William J. Clancy, Daniel J. Carey

Manifesto of Plain Facts

William J. Clancy, Daniel J. Carey

Manifesto of Plain Facts

ISBN/EAN: 9783743344679

Manufactured in Europe, USA, Canada, Australia, Japa

Cover: Foto ©ninafisch / pixelio.de

Manufactured and distributed by brebook publishing software (www.brebook.com)

William J. Clancy, Daniel J. Carey

Manifesto of Plain Facts

PREFACE.

IN INTRODUCING this Edition to the reader it would be only just and right to give an explanation as to how and why I came to do so.

Permit me to say, after I have had a number of years' practical experience in the manufacturing of preparations from animal product for the treatment of indigestion and dyspeptic symptoms, my attention was called to the medicinal properties of pepsin, its source and supply. I handled from 2,000 to 12,000 stomachs daily for four years. I received them in all stages, ranging in condition from the healthiest to the most disordered and inflamed, and I have never found any difference in the amount of pepsin contained therein or in quality, proportional to their weight; the poor animal and the fat being equally supplied, also the pancreas, though thinner and lighter in poor animals than in a fleshier and seemingly healthier one, always contained apparently an equal amount of the pancreatic juice and, having the same properties, being capable of converting equal weight of starch into sugar and emulsifying equal weight of fats. The animals, as a rule, were fed and housed alike, still there was a marked difference in their outward appearance and weight, and a greater difference in the composition of their blood and flesh. I found that the poor animal of same age as the sleek and fat one had nearly twice the amount of fluid blood, but of much lighter color, and only about one-half the amount of fibrin, the red blood corpuscles being much smaller, with very little difference in number.

The blood acid. I found in the lung cells of the poor animal flocks of coagulated blood from hameglobin, the lungs acting as a strainer and retaining all solid substance, upon microscopic examination of the flocks of coagulated hameglobin together with a careful chemical test, the flocks showed marked traces of carbonic acid gas, while the lungs were very much flattened and not of healthy color.

Following up this important discovery I concluded to make a special study of the disordered condition on general principals, selecting for my subject the sheep, and arrangements were made with the butchers to notify me when the government inspectors condemned cattle or sheep, which they did on a number of occasions, and I found a number of condemned animals suffering from the blight of tuberculosis. On microscopic examination I found the stomach in most cases contracted, the muscles and nerves dilated and in some parts solidified, while seeming to be almost devoid of plamsa, hence I came to the conclusion that tuberculosis is caused by a disordered condition of the stomach, inducing an abnormal blood supply with an ensuing impoverished nervous system, not containing the elements to produce activity, and that pulmonary tuberculosis is only a secondary trouble, while to successfully remove the bacilli and heal the lungs could only be accomplished by *treating the cause that was producing the trouble.* It is a well known fact that the lungs are a bacillicidal, and when properly supplied with motive or muscular power that by the air which they supply sufficient oxygen is taken in the blood to keep the red corpuscles up to highest possible point, and they in turn acting as we might say as the scavengers of the system, by giving up the oxygen, the life-giver, and absorbing in turn the carbonic gas and conveying it again to the lungs for exhalation, the chemical change takes place in the lungs, and carbonic with all obnoxous gasses are exhaled while a fresh supply of oxygen is partaken of, and so continues the work and action of the lungs. Understanding the normal lung function, they may be compared to a mechanical contrivance by way of comparison as a boiler generating steam, of which no use of it can be made until the steam is conveyed through pipes to radiators, where the heat is supplied, or again for motive power there is steam chest and cylinder; now, if for some reason the eccentric should be displaced so the cylinder could take steam from but one end, the force of power would be lost, and the machine would not move; now, in this case, with the engine at fault, if the engineer would say, " I must repair the boiler and raise more steam," what would you think of such a mechanic?

With the mechanism properly adjusted the machine will supply the required force and power; so it is with man, if the nervous system is supplied with the lacking elements they at once supply the muscles of the body with energy, and the muscles are then enabled to perform their respective functions, the lungs are compelled to respond to muscular contraction and the required amount of oxygen is supplied in the blood while obnoxious gasses are expelled, then the blood becomes healthy, as we know the blood is flesh—flesh is blood—and when the blood is healthy the tissues are also; nor if from any cause there is a breaking down or suppuration of tissue, the corpuscles will absorb the same as noxious gas, and convey it to the lung where it is expelled by the chemical action of the lung, and thus by combustion, in due time, the noxious poison is removed while healthy blood prevents its propagation by neutralization and the involved parts are healed.

We all recall the usual questions of many noted physicians to persons affected with pulmonary tuberculosis; the first question being, "How long have you been ailing?" "Have you reduced in flesh?" "Have you night-sweats?" "How is your appetite?" After examining the chest if in its incipiency, the physician will advise a bottle of "so-and-so" emulsion, take this and that, weigh yourself once each week, etc., etc., most invariably the patient will say: "Doctor, I am so nervous and irritable I can't sleep; can't you give me something? I believe if my stomach did not trouble me I would be all right." The cough at that time being only light, later on the cough becomes more aggravating and the stomach and nerves more upset, then the patient will call again and the physician will say to the patient: "When did you weigh last?" being told, "Have you gained any in weight?" "No, I have lost about three pounds each week notwithstanding that the most nutritious food has been partaken of." After examination the patient will ask the physician; "Well, doctor, what do you think of my case?" After a few moment's hesitancy the reply is: "I do not see much change in your lungs, and I am somewhat disappointed to learn that you have been losing in flesh and strength; now, let me see; how are you fixed financially? If it would be so that you could stand the expense I would advise you to go South," or West, as the case might be, "and take my medicine and rough it; you will be much improved." What are the results? about one chance in a hundred to regain his health, and twenty-five chances in one hundred to prolong his suffering for a few years at the most, and in no case have I ever seen where tubercular pulmonalis was cured by climatic treatment so the patients could return to their respective homes and enjoy *their cure*.

The physicians' trouble and failure in producing a cure in tubercular pulmonalis had for all time been the same; they have been treating the lungs some by inhilation, others by astringents drugs, such as creasote and oil of cloves, and have destroyed the action of the stomach, they have completely ignored the seat of the trouble, and treated the lungs, when, in fact, the lung symptoms are secondary.

The trouble with other so-called "*Consumption Cures*" has been the same in all cases; their originators started out with a false diagnosis, and were consequently led into errors in the treatment of the disease; upon the other hand, the success of my treatment of the disease is easily attributed to the fact that I have properly diagnosed the real cause of the disease, and went to work systematically upon these lines, and brought forth a specific which contains the missing elements of the nervous system. In other words: I found out what had to be cured, and studied out that *cure*.

This I was enabled to do on account of my wide experience in pharmaceutical chemistry and extensive knowledge of the pathological effects of the medicinal products in the manufacturing of which I was for years engaged. Having discovered a positive cure for consumption and kindred diseases, I concluded that a specific that would remove the cause and restore vitality would certainly not be injurious to be partaken of by persons in good health, I then decided to look for that patient, and finally I concluded that I myself would fill the bill. I immediately began to take the remedy, and continued to do so for three months, and I must say I experienced no bad results from its use. At that time I was 30 years of age, and never knew what it was to be sick. It is now eight years since, and my health is exceptionally good. Having satisfied myself that the medicine was not injurious to the system I then sought for persons who were afflicted with tuberculosis, and I found it to be a very difficult task to induce them to try the remedies while their attending physician held out any encouragement. Then, as a last resort, I concluded to try the remedies on a few cases that were far advanced—and, in fact, had given up all hopes—their physicians informed them or their friends that it was not necessary for the physician to call further, as all that could be done was accomplished, and to be kind and attentive to them as they would not live more than a week, or a month at the most. So I selected a number of such patients and treated them, and the results were so favorable that I cured fifty per cent. of those cases. Some of those are to-day well and following their usual occupations.

My theory of tuberculosis is a constitutional weakness and that if a cure is to be accomplished that it must be produced only by the increased vitality; hence, it was not proper for me to expect to cure a patient when their vitality was exhausted, as it is my firm conviction that medicine is only an assistant to nature to throw off the disease, and that no medicine cures of itself, but if properly and judiciously administered will assist nature and vitality to throw off the disease; hence the necessity of having a patient with a fair amount of vitality. A man's vitality can be compared to two horses heavily laden on a rough road that become exhausted and can't draw the load; man coming along with one horse says it represents medicine, and he will say: "Take off your horses and replace them with mine, *medicine*," do you believe that one will accomplish what two failed to? No, but if he places his horse's strength in connection with the other two the three will move along smoothly.

Through the kindness of a noted physician, who allowed me to test the medicine on two of his patients who were afflicted with tuberculosis of the lungs, and in second stage. After a few months' treatment they were pronounced cured and physically strong, and returned to their former occupations. During the treatment the attending physician noted their symptoms from day to day, also a number of physicians.

Shortly after, this physician said to me: " Clancy, what do you intend doing with the remedies?" My answer was, I would like to give the cure to the profession but that I was not financially able to, and, another reason, that it would require time to prove the effectiveness of the cure, and that I wished to personally superintend its administration, as a cure was at one time anticipated, when Dr. Koch said his cure was *perfect*, but when his so-called cured patients returned to work, they were without exception stricken down and died within the year, and I did not want to make an assertion unless I could substantiate the statement with positive cures—who had been cured for at least one year, and who were able to follow their usual occupation, also to live in any climate they chose.

This noted physician informed me that it would be necessary that I have a stock company incorporated under our State laws to administer the remedies only upon the prescription of duly qualified physicians, who should diagnose the patients' disease and prescribe it in proper cases.

I sought the advise of an attorney who was familiar with corporations law, also the ethics of medical profession. After selecting my associates, men of note, the application was presented to the department of State, State of Illinois. On the 1st day of July, 1896, a charter was granted for the organization of the ST. PHILLIP'S SPECIAL REMEDIES COMPANY. The remedies are since July 9, 1896, administered by the St. Phillip's Special Remedies Co. The Company is incorporated for ninety-nine years, and have the sole use of the remedies while the Company is in existence. The medicine is only given upon the prescription of qualified physicians, and in no case can the medicine be purchased outside the Company's laboratory, and in no case can it be purchased unless prescribed for. The medicine is *not for sale* in drug stores nor department stores.

Any physician can forward diagnosis blank giving symptoms and condition, and it in first or second stages would immediately fill the order. But if the patient is in the last stage, *would not* want to treat such patients, as we could not possibly hope for a *cure*.

The St. Phillip's Special Remedies Co. have in their Chicago office five regular physicians who make *examinations* and prescribe the treatment and administer to *any* and *all* complications that may *arise*.

I will now endeavor to call your attention to the physiological and chemical composition of the body, and if you carefully pursue it you will readily see that chemistry is the main factor, and if judiciously mastered will give the necessary light, so the cause can be located, also by close adherence to the grand and simple *leading truths* of chemistry, the lesser truths or principals, and nearly all the interesting relationships of elements and compounds. In a word, the science of chemistry must be dependent to bring out the specific to cure all ailments of man.

Read the book through carefully and note each testimonial, and I believe you will bear me out, and that we are the only Company, or body of men, that can produce *a positive cure* of that dread disease, viz: Consumption, and Bright's Disease.

We are desirous of having physicians interview us or our cured patients, or those under treatment. Also would be willing to supply the medicine to the profession in different localities, to be given gratuitiously, as on trial cases, providing a diagnosis is forwarded to our office, and the patient is not further advanced than second stage.

We maintain, we can positively cure ninety-eight per cent. of tuberculosis patients by the use of our remedies when in first stage, and at least seventy-five per cent. when in second; in third and last stage cannot cure them, but can relieve them and render the tubercular bacilli innocuous, so it cannot be propagated.

Bright's Disease can be cured in all of its stages. When uræmia is very marked, cannot cure them, but at any time before the blood is poisoned with urea can cure the disease; it makes no difference how much œdema is present.

CONTENTS.

CHAPTER I.
	PAGE.
Physiology, the Phenomena of Life	13
Heart and Liver	28
The Cell Nucleus	33
Structure of Protoplasmic Cells	35
The Body in Units	49

CHAPTER II.
Physiology of the Kidney	52
Physiology of the Nervous System	56
Circulation of the Blood	58
Secreting Cells	60
Vital Phenomena	71
Inhibition	78

CHAPTER III.
Bacilli of Tuberculosis	80

CHAPTER IV.
Essentials on Bacteriology	83

CHAPTER V.
Scrofula	95

CHAPTER VI.
Treatment of Scrofula	100

CHAPTER VII.
Pulmonary Tuberculosis	106

CONTENTS—(Continued.)

CHAPTER VIII.
	PAGE.
Cause of Pulmonary Tuberculosis	112

CHAPTER IX.
Pneumonia	116

CHAPTER X.
What Constitutes Bright's Disease	129
Acute Nephritis	132
Chronic Nephritis	134

CHAPTER XI.
Bright's Disease	138

CHAPTER XII.
Erythema	144

CHAPTER XIII.
Erysipelas	150

CHAPTER XIV.
General Diseases	156
Symptoms Acute Rheumatism	157
Heart Complications	159
Hydropathic Treatment	161
Muscular Rheumatism	163
Accessory Means	164
Chronic Rheumatism	165

CHAPTER XV.
Acute Gout	167
Difference between Gout and Rheumatism	170
Preventive Treatment	172
Chronic Gout	173

CHAPTER XVI.
Medical Journal of Health	176
Western Trade Journal	181

CONTENTS—(Continued.)

CHAPTER XVII.

	PAGE.
Inter Ocean	184
" "	189
Western Trade Journal	194
Catholic World	197

CHAPTER XVIII.

Hints on the Regulation of Diet	199
Relation of Food to Nutriment	202
Primary Use of Nitrogenous Food	205
Alcohol	207
Comparative Values of Animal Food	209
Fish and Oysters	213
Milk	215

CHAPTER XIX.

Vegetable Food	220
Fruits	231

CHAPTER XX.

Liquids	238
Ice	243

CHAPTER XXI.

Testimonials on Tuberculosis	247
" " Bright's Disease	281

CHAPTER I.

The word Physiology may be used either in a general or in a more restricted sense. In its more general meaning it was used largely of old, and is still occasionally used in popular writing, to denote all inquiry into the nature of living beings. A very slight acquaintance, however, with the phenomena of living beings shows that these can be studied from two apparently very different points of view.

The most obvious and striking character of a living being is that it appears to be an agent, performing actions and producing effects on the world outside itself. Accordingly the first efforts of inquirers were directed towards explaining how these actions are carried on, how the effects of a living being upon its surrounding are brought about. And the dissection or pulling to pieces of the material body of a living being was, under the name of Anatomy (q. v.) regarded as simply an analysis preparatory and necessary to the understanding of vital actions. But it soon became obvious that this anatomical analysis gave rise of itself to problems independent of, or having only distant relations to, the problems which had to do with the actions of living beings. Hence, in course of time a distinct science has grown up which deals exclusively with the laws regulating the form, external and internal, of living beings, a science which does not seek to explain the actions of living beings, and takes note of these actions only when they promise to throw light on the occurence of this or that structural feature. Such a science which is now known under the name of Morphology (*q. v.*) might be carried on in a world in which all living things had, in the ordinary meaning of the word, become dead. Were the whole world suddenly petrified or were a spell to come over it like that imagined by Tennyson in his Day Dream, but more intense, so that not only the gross visible movements but the inner invisible movements which are at the bottom of growth were all stayed, the morphologist would still find ample exercise for his mind in investigating the form and structure of the things which had been alive and which still differed from other things in their outward lineaments and internal build.

In its older sense physiology embraced these morphological problems and so corresponded to what is now called Biology (*q. v.*); in its more modern sense physiology leaves these matters on one side and deals only with the actions of living beings on their surrounding (the study of these necessarily involving the correlative study of the effect of the surrounding on the living being) and appeals to matters of form and structure only so far as they throw light on problems of actions. Looking forward into the far future we may perhaps dimly discern the day when morphology and physiology will again join hands, and all the phenomena of living beings both those which relate to form and those which relate to action will be seen to be the common outcome of the same molecular process. But that day is as yet most distant, and though occasionally even now the two sciences cross each other's path; action explaining form, and form in turn explaining action, the dominant ideas of the two are so distinct, the one from the other, that each must for a long time yet be developed along its own line. It is proposed to treat in the following pages of physiology in this narrower, more restricted sense.

If any one at the present day making use of the knowledge so far gathered in were to attempt a rough preliminary analysis of the phenomena of action of a living being, for instance, of one of the more complex so-called higher animals—such as man—he might proceed in some such way as the following:

One of the first, perhaps the first and most striking fact about man, is that he moves; his body moves of itself from place to place, and one part of the body moves on another. If we examine any one of these movements, such as the bending of the forearm on the arm, we find that it is brought about by certain masses of flesh called muscles, which from time to time contract—that is, shorten; and these muscles are so disposed that when they shorten and so bring their ends nearer together, certain bones are pulled upon and the arm is bent. Upon further examination it will be found that all the gross movements of the body, both the locomotion of the whole body and the movements of parts upon parts are carried out by the contraction or shortening of muscles. The muscles together with bones, tendons, and other structures, are arranged in various mechanical contrivances, many of them singularly complex; hence the great diversity of movements of which an animal or man is capable; but in all cases the central fact, that which supplies the motive power, is the contraction of a muscle, a shortening of its constituent fibres, whereby its two ends are brought for a while nearer together

When pursuing the analysis farther we attempt to solve the question: Why do muscles contract? We find that the muscles of the body are connected with what is called the central nervous system by certain strands of living matter called nerves; and we further find that, with some few exceptions which need not concern us now, the contractions of muscles are brought about by certain occult invisible changes called nervous impulses which travel along these nerves from the central nervous system to the muscles. Hence, when a nerve is severed the muscles to which the nerve belonged, thus cut adrift from the central nervous system, no longer stirred by impulses reaching it from thence, ceases to contract and remain motionless and, as it were, helpless. Pushing the problem still farther home, and asking how these impulses originate in the central nervous system, we find that this central nervous mass is connected, not only with the muscles by means of nerves which, carrying impulses outward from itself to the muscles, and so serving as instruments of movement, are called motor, or efferent nerves, but also with various surfaces and parts of the body by means of other nerves, along which changes or impulses travel inwards to itself in a centripetal fashion. Moreover, the beginnings or peripheral endings of these other nerves appear to be so constituted that various changes in the surrounding of the body, or internal changes in the body itself, give rise to impulses, which, thus originated, travel inwards to the central nervous system; hence, these nerves are spoken of as sensory or afferent. Such sensory impulses reaching the central nervous system may forthwith issue as motor impulses leading to movements; but on many occasions they tarry within the central mass, sweeping backwards and forwards along particular areas of its substance, thus maintaining for a while a state of molecular agitation and leading to movement at some subsequent period only. Moreover, we have reason to think that molecular disturbances may arise within the central nervous system apart from the advent, either past or present, of any impulses along sensory nerves. Lastly, the presence of these molecular agitations in the central nervous system whether the immediate result of some new afferent impulses or the much delayed and complicated outcome of some impulse which arrived long ago, or the product of internal changes apparently independent of all disturbance from without, and so far spontaneous, may be indicated by corresponding phases of what we speak of as consciousness. We are thus led to conceive of the central nervous system as, chiefly at least, the seat of a molecular turmoil maintained by multitudinous afferent impulses streaming in along the various afferent nerves, a turmoil which makes itself felt within as changes of consciousness, and produces effects without by movements wrought through motor nerves and muscles. And one large part of physiology has for its task the unraveling of the laws which govern this turmoil, which determine, in relation to the advent of afferent impulses and the occurrence of intrinsic changes, the issue of motor impulses, and thus the character of the resulting movements.

The movement of man or of an animal are not, however, the only salient facts of its existence.

Equally characteristic of him are the facts, (1) that he from time to time eats and must eat in order to live, and (2) that a supply of fresh air containing a certain quantity of oxygen is indispensable to his remaining alive. Viewed from a chemical point of view an animal body whether dead or alive, is a mass of complex unstable chemical substances, combustible in nature, *i. e.*, capable of being oxydized, and of being reduced by oxydation to simpler, more stable substances, with a setting free of energy. Combustible in the ordinary sense of the word an animal body is not by reason of the large excess of water which enters into its composition; but an animal body thoroughly dried will in the presence of oxygen burn like fuel, and, like fuel, give out energy as heat. The material products of that combustion are fairly simply consisting of water, carbonic acid, some amonia or nitrogen compounds, and a few salts. And these same substances appear also as the products of that slower combustion which we call decay; for whether the body be burnt swiftly in a furnace or rot away slowly in earth, air, or water, the final result is the same, the union of the complex constituent substance with the oxygen furnished from the air and their reduction thereby to the above-named products with a development of heat, which either, as in the first case, is rapid and appreciable, or, as in the second, is so slow and gradual as to be with difficulty recognized. Moreover, during life also the same conversion, the same oxydation, the same reduction of complex substances to simpler matters, the same setting free of energy present in the former, but absent in the latter, may be noted. The animal body dies daily, in the sense that at every moment some part of its substance is suffering decay, is undergoing combustion; at every moment complex substances full of latent energy are by process of oxydation reduced to simpler substances devoid of energy or containing but little.

This breaking down of complex substance, this continued partial decay, is indeed the source of the body's energy; each act of life is the offspring of an act of death. Each strain of muscle, every throb of the heart, all the inner work of that molecular turmoil of the nervous system of which we spoke above, as well as the chemical labor wrought in the many cellular laboratories of glands and membranes, every throw of the vital shuttle, means an escape of energy as some larger compacted molecule splits into smaller, simpler pieces. Within the body the energy thus set free bears many shapes, but it leaves the body in two forms alone, as heat and as the work done by the muscles of the frame. All the inner labor of the body, both that of the chemical gland-cells, of the vibrating nerve-substance, with its accompanying changes of consciousness, and of the beating heart and writhing visceral muscles, is sooner or later by friction, or otherwise, converted into heat; and it is as heat that the energy devolved in this labor leaves the body. Manifold as seems the body's energy it has but one sourse, the decay of living material, *i.e.*, the oxydation of complex substances diversely built up into various living matters, and but two ends—heat and muscular work. The continued setting free of energy which thus marks the living body, entailing as it does the continued breaking up and decay of living substance, constitutes a drain upon the body which must be met by constantly renewed supplies, or otherwise the body would waste away and its energy flicker out. Hence, the necessity on the one hand for that which we call food. which, however varied, is essentially a mixture of complex combustible energy holding bodies, and, on the other hand, for that other kind of food, which we call breath, and which supplies the oxygen whereby the complex oxydizable substance may be oxydized to simpler matters and their potential energy made to work. Thus food supplies the energy of the body, but in quantity *only*, not in *quality*. The food by itself, the dead food, can exhibit energy as heat only, with intervening phases of chemical action; before its energy can be turned into the peculiar groves of nervous and muscular action it needs to be transmuted into living substance, and in that transmutation there is a preliminary expenditure of part of the food's store of energy.

Here, then, we have a second view of physiological labor. To the conception of the body as an assemblage of molecular thrills—some started by an agent outside the body, by light, heat, sound, touch, or the like; others begun within the body, spontaneously as it were, without external cause; thrills which, traveling to and fro, mingling with and commuting each other, either end in muscular movements or die away within the body. To this conception we must add a chemical one that of the dead food continually being changed and raised into the living substance, and of the living substance continually breaking down into the waste matters of the body by processes of oxydation, and thus supplying the energy needed both for the unseen molecular thrills and the visible muscular movements.

Hence, the problems of physiology may in a broad sense be spoken of as threefold: (1) On the one hand, we have to search the laws according to which the complex unstable food is transmuted into the still more complex and still more unstable living flesh, and the laws according to which this living substance breaks down into simple stable waste products, void, or nearly void, of energy. (2) On the other hand, we have to determine the laws according to which the vibrations of the nervous substance originate from extrinsic and intrinsic causes, the laws according to which these vibrations pass to and fro in the body acting and reacting upon each other, and the laws according to which they finally break up and are lost, either in those swings of muscular contraction whereby the movements of the body are affected or in some other way. (3) And, lastly, we have to attack the abstruse problems of how these neural vibrations, often mysteriously attended with changes of consciousness, as well as the less subtle vibrations of the contracting muscles, are wrought out of the explosive chemical decompositions of the nervous and muscular substances, that is, of how the energy of chemical action is transmuted into and serves as the supply of that vital energy which appears as movement, feeling and thought.

Even a rough initial analysis however, such as we have just attempted to sketch, simple as it seems with our present knowledge, is an expression of an accumulated and corrected inquirers of many ages; the ideas which it embodies are the result of long continued investigations, and the residue of many successive phases of opinion.

In the natural hierarchy of the science physiology follows after chemistry, which in turn follows physics, molar and molecular; and in a natural developement, as indeed is evident from what we have just seen, the study of the two latter should precede that of the former. At a very early age, however, the exigencies of life brought the study of man, and so of physiology, to the front before its time; hence the history of physiology consists to a large extent, especially in its opening chapters, of premature vain attempts to solve physical and chemical problems before the advent of adequate physical or chemical knowledge. But no ignorance of these matters could hide from the observant mind, even in quite early times, two salient points which appear also in the analysis just given, namely, that, while some of the phenomena of living beings seem due to powers wholly unknown in things which are not living, other phenomena though at first sight special to living beings, appear to be in reality the peculiar outcome of processes taking place as well in things not alive. It was further early seen that while the former are much more conspicuous and make up a greater part of the life of the individual in those living beings which are called animals, especially in man, and in animals more closely resembling man, than in those which are called plants, the latter are common to both divisions of living things. Both sets of phenomena, however, were at first regarded as the products of certain special agencies, both were spoken of as the work of certain spirits; and the distinction between the two was formulated by speaking of the spirits as being in the former case animal, and in the latter vital.

From the very outset, even, the casual observer could not fail to be struck with the fact that many of the processes of living beings appear to be the results of the various contrivances or machines of which a living body is largely built up. This, indeed, was evident even before the distinction between animal and vital spirits was recognized; and when that differentiation was accepted, it was seen that the part played by these machines and contrivances in determining the actions of living beings was much more conspicuous in the domain of vital than of animal spirits. As inquiry was pushed forward the prominence and importance of this machinery became greater and greater, more especially since the phenomena supposes to be due to the agency of vital spirits proved more open to direct observation and experiment than those attributed to the animal spirits. It was found that the most fruitful path of investigation lay in the direction of studying the structure and independent action of the several constituent machines, of the body and of unravelling their mutual relations.

These machines received the names of organs, the work or action of an organ being at a later period spoken of as its function. And when it became clear that many of the problems concerned with what was supposed to be the work of the vital spirits could be solved by the proper appreciation of the functions of certain organs, it was inferred that the more difficult problems belonging to the animal spirits could be solved in the same way. Still later on it was found that the conception of organs and functions was not only quite separable from, but indeed antagonistic to, the hypothesis of the entiris called spirits.

In this way the first phase, as it may be called, of the science of physiology was evolved, a phase which lasted till quite recent times. Under this conception every living being, plant or animal, was regarded as a complex of organs, each with its respective function, as an engine built up of a number of intricately contrived machines, each performing its specific work. The whole animal body was parcelled out into organs, each of which was supposed to have its appropriate function; and the efforts of the investigation were directed, on the one hand, to a careful examination of the structural features of an organ with the view of determining by deduction what its function must be, and on the other hand, to confirming or correcting by observation and experiment the conclusions thus reached by the anatomical method. And the fruitfulness of this line of inquiry proved so great that the ideas directing it became absolutely dominant. In many cases the problem to be worked out was in reality a purely mechanical one. This was notably so in the great question of the circulation so brilliantly solved by Harvey. Putting aside for awhile the inquiry as to the origin of the force with which the walls of the heart press on the blood contained in the cavities, accepting the fact that the blood is thus pressed at each beat of the heart, all the other truths of the circulation which Harvey demonstrated are simply the outcome of certain mechanical conditions, such as the position and arrangement of the valves, the connection of various patent tubes, and the like. And many other problems, as, for instance, those connected with respiration, proved to be similarly capable of solution by the application of ordinary mechanical principles to anatomical facts.

So fruitful, and consequently so adequate, seemed this conception of living beings as built up of contrivances or organs, in contrast with the lifeless world in whose monotonous masses no such structural disposition could be recognized, that the word "organic" came into use as a term distinctive of living things. The phrase was especially adopted by the chemists, who for a long time classified their material into organic substances, *i. e.*, substance found only in living beings, and into inorganic substances, that is, substances occurring in lifeless bodies as well. Indeed, this nomenclature has not even yet been wholly abandoned. Triumphant, however, as was this mode of inquiry in these and similar instances, there remained in every investigation an unsolvable residue, like the question of the origin of force exerted by the heart referred to above, in speaking of Harvey's work; and in many other instances the questions which could not be solved on mechanical principles formed a great part of the whole problem. Thus in the case of the liver, careful dissection showed that minute tubes starting from all parts of the liver joined into one large canal, which opened into the small intestine, and observation and experiment taught that these tubes during life conveyed from the liver to the intestine a peculiar fluid called bile, which appeared on the one hand to originate in the liver, and, on the other, to be used up for some purpose in the intestine. But here the mere mechanical flow of the bile along the gall-ducts, instead of being of primary, was merely of secondary importance, and the problem of how the bile was generated and made its way into the small beginnings of the ducts was the greater part of the whole matter. This latter problem was left unsolved, and, indeed, for awhile unattempted. Nevertheless, the success in other directions attending the conception of organs and functions encouraged physiologists to speak of the liver as an organ whose function was to secrete bile, and, further, led them to ignore to a large extent the great unsolved portion of the problem, and to regard the mere enunciation of the function as the chief end of physiological inquiry. Moreover, whenever attempts were made to unravel these obscurer problems, the efforts of investigators were mainly confined to a fuller and more complete elucidation of the supposed function of an organ, and the method of inquiry adopted was in most cases one which regarded the finer elements of the part studied as minute organs making up the whole gross organ, and which sought to explain the functions of these smaller organs on the same mechanical principles which had proved so successful, in the case of the whole organ. When the improvements in the microscope opened up a new world to the anatomist, and a wholly fresh mechanical analysis of the structure of living bodies become possible, great hopes were entertained that the old method applied to the new facts would soon solve the riddles of life by showing how the mysterious operations of the living substances out of which the grosser organs were built were the outcome of structural arrangements which had hitherto remained invisible, were in fact the functions of minute component organs. A vision of a grand simplicity of organic nature dawned upon the minds of physiologists. It seemed possible to conceive of all living beings as composed of minute organic units, of units whose different actions resulted from their different structural characters, whose functions were explicable by, and could be deduced from their anatomical features, such units being built up into a number of gross organs, the functions of each of which could in turn be explained by the directions which its mechanical build gave to the efforts of its constituent units. Such a view seemed to have touched the goal when, in the first half of this century the so-called "cell theory" was enunciated as a physiological generalization.

It has long been a reproach to physiologists that, while to most organs of the body an appropriate function had been assigned, in respect to certain even conspicuous organs no special use or definite work could be proved to exist. Of these apparently functionless organs the most notorious instance was that of the spleen, a large and important body, whose structure, though intricate, gave no sign of what its labors were, and whose apparent uselessness was a stumbling-block to the theological speculations of Paley. While in the case of other organs a definite function could be readily enunciated in a few words, and their existence therefore easily accounted for, the spleen remained an opprobrium existing as it appeared to do, without purpose, and therefore without cause.

The progress of discovery during the present century was a cruel blow; instead of pointing out the missing use of the spleen, rudely shook the confidence with which the physiologists concluded that they had solved the riddle of an organ when they had allotted to it a special function.

From very old times it had been settled that the function of the liver was to secrete bile; and the only problems left for inquiry as touching the liver seemed to be those which should show how the minute structure of the organ was adapted for carrying on this work. About the middle of this century, however, the genius of Claud Bernard led him to the discovery that the secretion of bile was by no means the chief labor of the liver. He showed that this great viscus had other work to do than that of secreting bile, had another function to perform but a function which seemed to have no reference whatever to the mechanical arrangements of an organ, which could never have been deduced from any inspection, however complete of its structure, even of its most hidden and minute features and which, therefore, could not be called a function in the old and proper sense of that word. By a remarkable series of experiments which might have been carried out by one knowing absolutely nothing of the structural arrangements of the liver, beyond the fact that blood flowed to it along the portal vein, and from it along the hepatic vein, he proved that the liver, in addition to the task of secreting bile, was during life engaged in carrying on a chemical transformation by means of which it was able to manufacture and store up in its substance a peculiar kind of starch, to which the name of glycogen was given. Bernard himself spoke of this as the glycogenic function of the liver, but he used the word "function" in a broad, indefinite sense, simply as work done, and not in the older, narrower meaning as work done by an organ structurally adapted to carry on a work which was the inevitable outcome of the form and internal build of the organ. In this glycogenic function organization, save only the arrangements by means of which the blood flows on from the portal to the hepatic channels in close proximity to the minute units of the liver substance, the so-called hepatic cells appear to play no part whatever; it was not a function, and in reference to it the liver was not an organ in the old sense of the word. This discovery of Bernard's threw a great flash of light into the darkness hitherto hiding the many ties which bound together distant and mechanically isolated parts of the animal body. Obviously the liver made this glycogen, not for itself, but for other parts of the body; it labored to produce, but they made use of the precious material, which thus became a bond of union between the two.

The glycogenic labors of the simple hepatic substance carried out independently of all intricate structural arrangements, and existing in addition to the hepatic function of secreting bile being thus revealed, men began to ask themselves the question: May not something like this be true of other organs to which we have allotted a function, and thereupon rested content? And, further, in the case where we have striven in hope, and yet in vain, to complete the interpretation of the function of an organ by finding in the minute microscopic details of its structure the mechanical arrangements which determine its work, may not have followed throughout a false lead, and sought for organization where organization in our sense of the word does not exist? The answer to this question, and that an affirmative one, was hastened by the collapse of the cell theory on his physiological side very soon after it had been distinctly formulated.

The cell, according to the views of those who first propounded the cell theory, consisted essentially of an envelope, or cell membrane of a substance contained within the cell membrane, hence called cell contents, and of a central body or kernel called the "nucleus," differing in nature from the rest of the cell contents. And when facts were rapidly accumulated all tending to prove that the several parts of the animal or vegetable body, diverse as they were in appearance and structure, were all built up of cells more or less modified

The hope arose that the functions of the cell might be deducted from the mutual relations of cell membrane, cell contents, and nucleus, and that the functions of an organ might be deduced from the modified functions of the constituent modified cells. Continued investigation, however, proved destructive of this physiological cell theory.

It soon became evident that the procession of an investing envelope or cell membrane was no essential feature of a cell, and that even the central kernel or nucleus might at times be absent. It was seen in fact that the anatomical unit need have no visible parts at all, but might be simply a minute mass, limited in various ways, of the material spoken of as cell contents. Under the cell theory the cell was supposed to be the first step in organization, the step by which a quantity of a formless unorganized plasm became an organized unit; this plasm was further supposed still to form the chief part of the cell contents, and soon became recognized under the name of protoplasm. Hence the destructive anatomical researches which deprived the cell of its cell membrane, and even of its uucleus, left nothing except a mass of protoplasm to constitute an anatomical unit. For such unit the word "cell" was a misnomer, since all the ideas of organization denoted by the word had thus vanished; nevertheless it was retained with the new meaning, and up to the present time the definition of a cell is that of a limited mass of protoplasm, generally, but not always, containing a modified kernel or nucleus.

With this anatomical change of front the physiological cell theory was utterly destroyed. The cell was no longer a unit or organization; it was merely a limited mass of protoplasm, in which beyond the presence of a nucleus, there was no visible distinction of parts. It was no longer possible to refer the physiological phenomena of the cell to its organization it became evident that the work done by a "cell" was the result not of its form and cellular structure, but simply of the nature and properties of the apparently structureless protoplasm which formed its body. A new idea pressed itself on men's minds, that organization was a concomitant and result of vital action, not its condition and cause as Huxley in one of his earliest writings put it, "They (cells) are no more the producers of the vital phenomena than the shells scattered in ordinary lines along the sea-beach are the instruments by which the gravitative force of the moon acts upon the ocean. Like these the cells mark only where the vital tides have been, and how they have acted." Hence, arose the second of the two movements mentioned above, that which may be called the protoplasmic movements, a movement which throwing overboard altogether all conceptions of life as the outcome of organization, as the mechanical result of structural conditions, attempts to put physiology on the same footing as physics and chemistry, and regards all vital phenomena as the complex products of certain fundamental properties exhibited by matters, which either from its intrinsic nature or from its existing in peculiar conditions, is known as living matter, mechanical contrivances in the form of organs serving only to modify in special ways the results of the exercise of these fundamental activities and in no sense determining their initial developements.

Long before the cell theory had reduced to an absurdity the "organic" conception of physiology, the insight of the brilliant Bichat, so early lost to science, had led him to prepare the way for modern views by developing his doctrine of tissue. That doctrine regarded the body as made up of a number of different kinds of living material, each kind of material having certain innate qualities proper to itself as well as certain structural features, and the several kinds of material being variously arranged in the body. Each of these body components was spoken of as a tissue, muscular tissue, nervous tissue and the like; and the varied actions of the body were regarded as the result of the activities of the several tissues modified and directed by the circumstances that the tissues were to a great extent arranged in mechanical contrivances or organs which largely determine the character and scope of their action.

The imperfection of microscopic methods in Bichat's time, and we may perhaps add, his early death, prevented him from carrying out an adequate analysis of the qualities or properties of the tissues themselves. During the middle portion of this century, however, histological investigation, *i. e.*, inquiry into the minute structure of the tissues, made enormous progress, and laid the bases for a physiological analysis of the properties of tissues. In a short time it became possible to lay down the generalization that all the several tissues arise, as far as structure is concerned, by a differentiation of a simple primitive living matter and that the respective properties of each tissue are nothing more than certain of the fundamental properties of the primordial substance thrown into prominence by a division of labor running to a certain extent parallel to the differentiation of structure. Developed in a fuller manner this modern doctrine may be expounded somewhat as follows:

In its simplest form, a living being, as illustrated by some of the forms spoken of as *amocbæ*, consists of a mass of substance in which there is no obvious distinction of parts. In the body of such a creature even the highest available powers of the microscope reveal nothing more than a fairly uniform network of material, a network sometimes compressed, with narrow meshes, sometimes more open, with wider meshes, the intervals of the meshwork being filled, now with a fluid, now with a more solid substance or with a finer and more delicate network, and minute particles or granules of variable size being sometimes lodged in the open meshes, sometimes deposited in the strands of the network. Sometimes, however, the network is so close, or the meshes filled up with material so identical in refractive power with the bars or films of the network, and at the same time so free from granules, that the whole substance appears absolutely homogeneous, glassy or hyaline. Analysis with various staning and other reagents leads to the conclusion that the substance of the network is of a different character from the substance filling up of the meshes. Similar analysis shows that at times the bars or film of the network are not homogeneous, but composed of different kinds of stuff; yet even in these cases it is difficult if not impossible to recognize any definite relation of the components to each other such as might deserve the name of structure; and certainly in what may be taken as the more typical instance where the network seems homogeneous, no microscopic search is able to reveal to us a distinct structural arrangement in its substance. In all probability optical analysis, with all its aids, has here nearly reached its limit; and, though not wholly justified, we may perhaps claim the right to conclude that the network in such case is made up of a substance in which no distinction of parts will ever be visible, though it may vary in places or at times

in what may be spoken of as molecular construction, and may carry, lodged in its own substance a variety of matters foreign to its real self. This remarkable network is often spoken of as consisting of protoplasm, and though that word has come to be used in several different meanings, we may for the present retain the term. The body of an *amoeba*, then, or of a similar organism consists of a network or framework which we may speak of as protoplasm, filled up with other matters. In most cases it is true that in the midst of this protoplasmic body there is seen a peculiar body of a somewhat different and yet allied nature, the so-called nucleus; but this we have reason to think is specially concerned with processes of division or reproduction and may be absent, for a time at all events, without any inquiry to the general properties of the protoplasmic body.

Now, such a body, such a mass of simple protoplasm, homogeneous save for the admixtures spoken of above, is a living body, and all the phenomena which I sketched out at the beginning of this article as characteristic of the living being may be recognized in it. There is the same continued chemical transformation, the same rise and fall, in chemical dignity, the same rise of the dead food into the more complex living substance, the same fall of the living substance into simpler waist products. There is the same power of active movement, a movement of one part of the body upon another giving rise to a change of form, and a series of changes of form resulting eventually in a change of place. In what may be called the condition of rest the body assumes a more or less spherical shape. By the active transference of part of the mass in this or that direction the sphere flattens itself into a disk, or takes on the shape of a pear, or of a rounded triangle, or assumes a wholly irregular, often a star-shaped or branched form. Each of these transformation is simply a rearrangement of the mass without change of the bulk. When a bulging of one part of the body takes place there is an equivalent retraction of some other part or parts; and it not unfreqently happens that one part of the body is repeatedly thrust forward, bulging succeeding bulging, and each bulging accompanied by a corresponding retraction of the opposite side so that by a series of movements the whole body is shifted along the line of the protuberance. The tiny mass of simple living matters move onward, and that with some rapidity, by what appears to be a repeated flux of its simi-liquid substance.

The internal change leading to these movements may begin, and the movements themselves to be executed, by any part of the uniform body, and they may take place without any obvious cause. So far from being always the mere passive result of the action of extrinsic forces they may occur spontaneously, that is, without the coincidence of any recognizable disturbance whatever in the external condition to which the body is exposed, they appear to be analogous to what in higher animal we speak of as acts of volition. They may, however, be provoked by changes in the external conditions. A quiescent *amobæ* may be excited to activity by the touch of some strange body, or by some other event, by which in the ordinary language of phisiology is spoken of as a *stimulus*. The protoplasmic mass is not only mobile but sensitive. When a stimulus is applied to one part of the surface a movement may commence in another and quite distinct part of the body; that is to say, molecular disturbances appear to be propagated along its substance without visible change, after the fashion of the nervous impulses we spoke of in the beginning of this article. The uniform protoplasmic mass of the *amobæ* exhibits the rudiments of those attributes of powers which in the initial sketch we describe as being the fundamental characteristics of the muscular and nervous structures of the higher animals.

These facts and other considerations which might be brought forward lead to the tentative conception of protoplasm as being a substance (if we may use that word in a somewhat loose sense) not only unstable in nature but subject to incessant change, existing indeed as the expression of incessant molecular, that is chemical and physical change, very much as a fountain is the expression of an incessant replacement of water. We may picture to ourselves this total change which we denote by the term "metabolism" as consisting on the one hand of a downward series of changes (katabolic change) a stair of many steps, in which more complete bodies are broken down with the setting free of energy into simpler waste bodies, and, on the other hand, of an upward series of changes, (anabolic change), also a stair of many steps, by which the dead food of varying simplicity or complexity is, with the further assumption of energy, built up into more and more complex bodies. The summit of this double stair we call "protoplasm." Whether we have a right to speak of it as a single body, in the chemical sense of that word, or as a mixture in some way of several bodies, whether we should regard it as the very summit of the double stair or as embracing as well the topmost steps on either side, we cannot at present tell. Even if there be a single substance forming the summit, its existence is absolutely temporary; at one instance it is made, at the next it is unmade. Matter which is passing through the phase of life rolls up the ascending steps to the top and forthwith rolls down on the other side. But to this point we shall return later on. Further, the dead food, itself fairly but far from wholly stable in character, becomes more and more unstable as it rises into the more complex living material. It becomes more and more explosive, and when it reaches the summit its equilibrium is overthrown and it actually explodes. The whole downward stair of events seems in fact to be a series of explosions, by means of which the energy latent in the dead food and augumented by the touches through which the dead food becomes living protoplasm is set free. Some of this freed energy is used up again within the material itself, in order to carry on this same vivification of dead food; the rest leaves the body as heat or motion. Sometimes the explosions are, so to speak, scattered going off, as it were, irregularly throughout the material like a quantity of gunpowder sprinkled over a surface, giving rise to innumerable minute puffs, but producing no massive visible effects. Sometimes they take place in unison, many occurring together, or in such rapid sequence that a summation of their effects is possible, as in gunpowder rammed into a charge, and we are then able to recognize their result as visible movements or as appreciable rise of temperature.

These various phenomena of protoplasm may be conveniently spoken of under the designation of so many properties or attributes, or powers of protoplasm, it being understood that these words are used in a general and not in any definite scholastic sense. Thus we may speak of protoplasm as having the power of assimilation, *i. e.*, of building up the dead food into its living self; of movement or of contractility as it is called, *i. e.*, of changing its form through internal explosive changes; and of irritability or sensitiveness, *i. e.*, of responding to external changes, by less massive internal explosions which spreading through its mass, are not in themselves recognizable through visible changes, though they may initiate the larger visible changes of movement.

These and other fundamental characters, all associated with the double upward and downward series of chemical changes of constructive and destructive metabolism, are present in protoplasm wherever found, but a very brief survey soon teaches us that specimens of protoplasm existing in different beings or in different parts of the same differ widely in the relative prominence of one or another of these fundamental characters. On the one hand, in one specimen of protoplasm the energy which is set free by the series of explosions constituting the downward changes of destructive metabolism may be so directed as to leave the mass almost wholly in the form of heat, thus producing very little visible massive change of form. Such a protoplasm consequently, however, irritable and explosive, exhibits little power of contractility or movement. In another specimen on the other hand, a very large portion of the energy similarly set free may be spent in produing visible changes of form, the protoplasm in this instance being exquisitely mobile. Such difference must be due to different internal arrangements of the protoplasm, though since no vision, however well assisted, can detect these arrangements, they must be of a molecular nature rather than of that grosser kind which we generally speak of as structural. It is true that as the difference in properties become more and more prominent, as the protoplasm becomes more and more specialized, features which we can recognize as structural intervene; but even these appear to be subsidiary to accompany and to be the result of the differences in property, or to be concerned in giving special directions to the activities developed, and not to be the real cause of the differences in action. We are thus led to the conception of protoplasm as existing in the various differentiated conditions while still retaining its general protoplasmic nature, a difference of constitution making itself felt in the different character of the work done, in a variation of the results of the protoplasmic life. We have a division of physiological labor going hand in hand with a differentiation of material, accompanied ultimately by morphological results which may be fairly spoken of as constituting a differentiation of structure.

Some of the simpler and earlier features of such a division and differentiation may be brought out by comparing with the life of such a being as the *amoebæ* that of a more complex and yet simple osganism as the *hydra* or fresh water *polyp*. Leaving out certain details of structure, which need not concern us now, we may say that the *hydra* consists of a large number of units or cells firmly attached to each other, each cell become composed of protoplasm, and its broad features resembling *amocbœ*. The *polyp* is in fact a group or crowd of *amocbœ*-like cells so associated together that not only may the material of each cell, within limits, be interchanged with that of neighboring cells, but also the dynamic events taken place in one cell, and leading to exhibitions of energy, may be similarly communicated to neighboring cells, also within limits. These cells are arranged in a particular way to form the walls of a tube of which the body of the *hydra* practically consists. They form two layers in apposition, one an internal layer called the *endoderm*, lining the tube, the other an external layer called the *ectoderm*, forming the outside of the tube. And putting aside minor details, the differences in structure and function observable in the organism are confined to differences between the *ectoderm* on the one hand, all the constituent cells of which are practically alike, and the *endoderm* on the other, all the cells of which are in turn similarly alike. The protoplasm of the *ectoderm* cells is so constituted as to exhibit in a marked degree the phenomena of which we spoke above as irritavility and contractility, whereas in the *endo-*

derm these phenomena are in abeyance, those of assimilation being prominent. The movements of the *hydra* are chiefly brought about by changes of form of the *ectoderm* cells, especially of tail-like process of these cells, which, arranged as a longitudinal wrapping of the tubular body, draw it together when they shorten, and lengthen it out when they elongate, it is by the alternate lengthening and shortening of its body, and of the several parts of its body, that the *hydra* changes its form and moves from place to place. Inaugurating these changes of form, the products of contractility are the more hidden changes of irritability; these also are especially developed in the *ectoderm* cells, and travel readily from cell to cell, so that a disturbance originating in one cell, either from some extrinsic cause, such as contact with a foreign body or from intrinsic events, may sweep from cell to cell over the surface of the whole body. The animal feels as well as moves by means of its *ectoderm* cells. In the *endoderm* cells the above phenomena, though not wholly absent, are far less striking, for these cells are almost wholly taken up in the chemical work of digestion and assimilating the food received into the cavity, the lining of which they form.

Thus the total labor of the organism is divided between these two membranes. The *endoderm* cells receive food, transmute it, and prepare it in such a way that it only needs a few final touches to become living material, these same cells getting rid at the same time of useless ingredients and waste matter. Of the food thus prepared the *endoderm* cells, however, themselves use but little; the waste of substance involved in the explosions which carry out movement and felling is reduced in them to a minimum; they are able to pass on the greater part of the alaborated nourishment to their brethren, the *ectoderm* cells. And these thus amply supplied with material which it needs but little expenditure of energy on their part to convert into their living selves, thus relieved of the greater part of nutritive labor are able to devote nearly the whole of their energies to movement and to feeling.

Microscopic examinations further shows that these two kinds of cells differ from each other to some extent in visible characters; and though, as we have seen, the differences in activity appear to be dependent on differences in invisible molecular arrangement rather than on gross visible differences such as may be called structural, still the invisible differences involve or entail, or are accompanied by visible differences, and such differences as can be recognized between *endoderm* and *ectoderm*, even with our present knowledge may be correlated to difference in their work; future inquiry will probably render the correlation still more distinct.

The foregoing rough analysis leads to a conception of physiology of the animal body may be expressed somewhat as follows:

The body is composed of different kinds of matter; each kind of matter, arranged in units more or less discrete, constitutes a tissue; and the several tissues, though having a common likeness in token of their origin from a common primordial protoplasm, have dissimilar molecular constitutions entailing dissimilar modes of activity. Nor is each tissue homogeneous for two parts of the body, though so far alike as to be both examples of the same general tissue, may be a different in molecular constitution, more or less distinctly expressed by microscopic difference of structure, and correspondingly different in action. Thus a liver cell and a kidney cell, though both examples of grandular tissue, are quite distinct, so also several varieties of muscular tissue exist; and in the dominant nervous tissue we have not only a broad distinction between nerve fibres and nerve cells, but the several groups of nerve cells which are built up into the brain and spinal cord, and, indeed, probably the single nerve cells of these, though all possessing the general characters both in structure and function, of nervous protoplasm, differ most widely from each other. These several tissues of diverse constitution and activity ranging as regards the rapidity of the molecular changes taken place in them from the irritable unstable, swiftly changing nerve cell, to the stable, slowly changing almost lifeless tendon or bone are disposed in the body in various mechanical arrangements constituting organs or machines, whereby the activities of the constituent tissue elements are brought to bear in special directions. These organs range from those in which the mechanical provisions are dominant, the special activity of the tissue elements themselves being in the background and supplying only an obscure or even unimportant factor, as in the organs of respiration, to those in which the mechanical provisions are insignificant, as in the central nervous system, where the chief mechanical factor is supplied by the distribution in space of the nerve fibres or cells.

Hence, it is obvious that almost every physiological inquiry of any large scope is, or sooner or later, becomes a mixed nature. On the one hand investigation has to be directed to the processes taking place in the actual tissue elements, in the protoplasmic cells and modifications of cells. These are essentially of a molecular, often of a chemical or chemico-physical nature, in the problems thus raised matters of form and structure, other than that of molecular structure which no microscope can ever reveal, and are of secondary moment only, or have no concern in the matter at all. These may be spoken of as the purely physiological or as the molecular problems. On the other hand, the natural results of these tissue activities are continually being modified by circumstances whose effect can be traced to the mechanical arrangements under which the tissue in question is acting, whence arise problems which have to be settled on simple mechanical principles.

CHAPTER II.

We may take as an illustration the physiology of the kidney. In the old language the function of the kidney is to secrete urine. When we come to inquiry into the matter, we find in the first place that the secretion of urine, that is, the quantity and quality of the urine escaping from the duct of the kidney in a given period, is partly determined by the quantity of blood passing through the kidney and the circumstances of its passage. Now, the quantity of blood reaching the kidney at any one time is dependent partly on the width of the renal arteries, partly on the general pressure of the blood in the arterial system. The width of the renal arteries is in turn dependent on the condition of their muscular walls, whether contracted or relaxed; and this condition is determined by the advent of nervous impulses, the so-called vaso-motor impulses arising in the central nervous system and passing down to the renal arteries along certain nerves. The emission of these vaso-motor impulses from the central nervous system is further determined, on the one hand by the condition of certain parts of the central nervous system, the so-called vaso-motor centres, and on the other by the passage of certain afferent sensory impulses to those vaso-motor centres from sensory surface such as the skin. Similarly the general blood pressure is dependent on the condition, patent or narrowed of the small arteries generally, this being likewise governed by the vaso-motor system and on the coincident work done by the heart in driving blood into the great blood vessels, this work being also governed by the nervous system. Hence, in attacking such a problem as to how any particular event, such as the exposure of skin to the cold, influences the flow of blood through the kidney and thus the secretion of urine, the investigator, without staying to inquire into the nature of nervous impulses, or into the nature of changes taking place in vaso-motor centres, etc., directs his attention to determining what impulses are generated under the circumstances, what paths they take, to what extent they are quantitively modified, how far they and their effects reach upon each other, and so on. His inquiry in fact takes on to a large extent the characters of an attempt to unravel an intricate game in which the counters are nervous impulses, muscular contractions and elastic reactions, but in which the moves are determined by topographical distribution and mechanical arrangements.

But there are other problems connected with the physiology of the kindey of quite a different nature. The kidney is, broadly speaking, constructed of living protoplasmic cells so arranged that each cell is on one side bathed with blood and lymph, and on the other forms the boundary of a narrow canal, which, joining with other canals, ultimately opens into the urinary bladder. Here the question arises how it is that these protoplasmic cells, having nothing to draw upon but the common blood which is distributed to other organs and tissues as well, are able to discharge on the other side of them into the canal the fluid urine, which is absolutely distinct from blood, which contains substance wholly unknown in blood, as well as substances which, though occurring in blood, are found there in minute quantities only, and, moreover, are not found to escape from the blood into any other tissues or organs. In attempting to answer this question we come upon an inquiry of quite different nature from the preceding, an inquiry for the solution of which mechanical suggestions are useless. We have to deal here with the molecular actions of the protoplasmic cells. We must seek for molecular explanations of the questions why a current sets across the cells from blood capillary and lymph space to the hallow canal; why the substances which emerge on the far side are so wholly unlike those which enter in or near the side, why, moreover, the intensity of this current may wax and wane now flooding the canal with urine, now nearly or quite drying up; why not only the intensity of the current but also the absolute and relative amount of the chemical substances carried along it are determined by events taking place in the cell itself, being largely independent of both the quantity and quality of the blood which forms the cells' only source of supply. These and other like questions can only be solved by looking with the mind's eye, by penetrating through careful inferences into those inner changes which we call molecular, and which no optical aid will ever reveal to the physical eye.

The master tissues and organs of the body are the nervous and muscular system, the latter being, however, merely the instrument to give effect and expression to the motions of the former. All the rest of the body serves simply either in the way of mechanical aids and protections to the several parts of the muscular and nervous system, or as a complicated machinery to supply these systems with food and oxygen, *i. e.*, with blood, and to keep them cleansed from waste matters throughout all their varied changes. The physiology of the muscular system is fairly simple. The mechanical problems involved have been long ago for the most part worked out, and the molecular problems which touch on the nature of muscular contractions, their dependence on the blood supply, and their relations to nervous impulses are being rapidly solved. The physiology of the nervous system, on the other hand, is in its infancy. The mechanical side of inquiry is here represented, inasmuch as the various actions of the system are conditioned by the distribution and topographical arrangement of the constituent fibres and cells; and even these simple problems, as may be seen from the article "Nervous System" below, are as yet largely unworked. The deeper molecular problems, those which deal with the real nature of the processes taking place in cell and fibre, even the simpler of these, such as the one which asks why the neural protoplasm of one cell, or group of cells, seems quiescent until stirred by some foreign impulse its own vibrations being otherwise retained and lost within its own substance, while the neural protoplasm of another cell is continually, or from time to time, discharging vibrations, as rythmic molecular pulses, along adjoining fibres, these at the present day can hardly be said to be touched. The physiology of the nervous system is emphatically the physiology of the future.

The rest of the body may, from a broad point of view, be regarded as a complex machinery for supplying these master tissues with adequately prepared food and oxygen, for cleansing them from the waste products of their activity and for keeping them at a temperature suitable for the development of their powers. As we have already said, the blood is the agent which not only supplies both food and oxygen but sweeps away all refuse and, we may add, is the instrument for maintaining an adequate temperature. All the rest of the body may in fact be looked upon as busied in manufacturing food into blood, in keeping up the oxygen supply of the blood, in sifting out from the blood all waste material, and in maintaining the blood at a uniform heat. This work, of which blood is, so to speak, the centre, is, as we have already seen, carried out by protoplasmic cells, many of which are themselves of a muscular nature, often forming part of complicated mechanical contrivances, built up partly of inert tissues, partly of active tissues, such as muscle and nerve. In tracing the food and oxygen into the blood and the waste matters out of the blood, in studying the distribution of the blood itself and the means adopted to maintain its even temperature, we come, as before, on problems partly mechanical or chemical and partly molecular. The changes which the food undergoes in the intestine can be, and have been, successfully studied as a series of purely chemical problems conditioned by anatomical arrangements, such as the existence of an acid fluid in the stomach, succeeded by alkaline fluids in the intestine, and the like; but the question concerned in the discharge of the digestive juices into the ailmentary canal, in the secretary activity of the digestive glands, raise up protoplasmic molecular inquiries. In the reception or absorption of the digested food we similarly find the purely physical process of diffesion and the like overriden by the special protoplasmic activities of the constituent cells of the lining of the canal.

In the further elaboration of the digested products the action of cells again intervenes, as it similarly does in the, so to speak, inverted action by which waste matters are cast out of the body though in both cases the results are in part conditioned by mechanical contrivances.

The circulation of the blood is carried on by means of an intricate mechanical contrivance, whose working is determined and whose effects are conditioned by molecular changes occurring in the constituent muscles and other protoplasmic cells; the work done by the heart, the varying width of the channels, the transit of material through the filmy capillary walls, all these are at once the results of protoplasmic activity and factors in the mechanical problems of the flow of blood. The oxygen passes into and carbonic acid out of the blood, through simple diffusion, by means of the respiratory pump, which is merely a machine whose motive power is supplied by muscular energy, and both oxygen and carbonic acid are carried along in the blood by simple chemical means; but the passage of oxygen from the blood into the tissue and of carbonic acid from the tissue into the blood, though in themselves mere diffusion processes, are determined by the molecular activity of the constituent cells of the tissue. Lastly, the blood, however well prepared, however skillfully driven to the tissue by the well-times activity of the vascular system, even when it has reached the inner network of the tissue elements is not as yet the tissue itself. To become the tissue it must undergo molecular changes of the profoundest kind, it must cross boundary from dead material to living stuff. The ultimate problems of nutrition are of the molecular kind. All the machinery, however elaborate, is preparatory only, and it is the last step which costs most.

Of the many problems concerned in these several departments of physiology the one class which we have spoken of as being mechanical in nature is far too varied to be treated of as a whole. The problems falling under it have but few features in common; each stands, as it were, on its own bottom, and has to be solved in its own way. The problems of the other class, however, those which we have spoken of as being molecular in nature, have a certain common likeness, and it may be worth while to consider in a brief and general manner some of their most striking characters.

For this purpose we may first of all turn to the changes taking place in a secreting cell, for these have of late years been studied with signal success. They illustrate what may be called the chemical aspects of vital actions, just as the changes in a muscular fibre, on the other hand, seem to present in their simplest forms, the kinetic aspects, of the same action. If we examine a secreting gland, such as a pancreas or a salivary gland, we find it is composed of a number of similar units, the unit being a secreting cell of approximately spheroidal form, one part of the surface of which borders a canal continuous with the duct of the gland, while another part is bathed in lymph. The process of secretion consists in the cell discharging into the canal a fluid which is of a sepecific character insomuch as, though it consists partly of water and other substances common to it and other fluid of the body, these are present in it in special proportions; and it also contains substances or a substance found in itself and nowhere else. To enable it to carry on this work the cell receives supplies of material from the lymph in which it is bathed, the lymph in turn being replenished from neighboring capillary blood vessels. The secreting cell itself consists of a soft protoplasmic "body" of the nature previously described in the midst of which lies a nucleus. The consideration of the actions carried out by the nucleus may for simplicity's sake be left on one side for the present; and may regard the cell as a mass of protoplasm consisting, as we have seen, of a network of a particular nature, and of other substances of different nature filling up the meshes or intersticies of the network.

Such a cell may exist under two different conditions. At one time it may be quiescent; although the blood vessels surrounding it are bathing it with lymph, although this lymph has free access to the protoplasm of the cell, no secretion takes place, no fluid whatever passes from the cell into the canal which it borders. At another time, under, for instance, some influence reaching it along the nerve distributed to the glands, although there may be no change in the quantity or quality of the blood passing through the adjacent blood vessels, a rapid stream of material flows from the protoplasmic cell body in the canal. How is this secretion brought about?

If we examine certain cells, such, for instance, as those of the pancreas, we find that during a period of rest succeeding one of activity the cell increases in bulk, and, further, that the increase is not so much an enlargement of the protoplasmic network as an accumulation of material in the meshes of the network; in fact there appears to be a relative diminution of the actual protoplasm, indicating, as we shall see, a conversion of the substance of the network into the material which is lodged in the interstices of the network. This material may and frequently does exist in the form of discrete granules recognizable under the microscope; and in the pancreas there is a tendency for these granules to be massed together on the side of the cell bordering the lumen of the canal. During activity while the cell is discharging its secretion into the canal these granules disappear so that the protoplasmic network is after prolonged activity left with a very small burden of material in its meshes; at the same time there also appears to be an accompanying absolute increase of growth of the mass of the protoplasm itself. We have further evidence that the substance which is thus stored up in the meshes of the cell forming the granules for instance just spoken of, is not, as it exists in the cells, the same substance as that which occurs in the secretion as its characteristic constituent. Thus the characteristic constituent of pancreatic juice is a peculiar ferment body called "trypsin" and we possess evidence that the granules in the pancreatic cells are not trypsin. But we have evidence also that these granules consist of material which upon a very slight change becomes trypsin of material which is antecedent of trypsin and which has accordingly been called trypsinogen. Thus the cell during rest stores up trypsinogen, and the change which characterizes activity is the conversion of trypsinogen into trypsin and its consequent discharge from the cell. These facts are ascertained by observation and experiment, viz: that trypsinogen appears in the protoplasm of the cell, and that in the act of secretion this trypsinogen is discharged from the cell in the form of the simpler trypsin. When, however, we come to consider the origin of the trypsinogen we pass to matters of inference and to a certain extent of speculation.

Two views seem open to us. On the one hand we may adopt an old theory, once generally accepted, and suppose that the cell picks out from the lymph which bathes it particles of typsinogen, or particles of some substance which is readily transformed into trypsinogen, and deposits them its substance. This may be called the "selective" theory. On the other hand, we may suppose that the trypsinogen results from the breaking down from the katabolic or destructive metabolism of the protoplasm being thus wholly formed in the cell. This may be called the "metabolic" theory. Our present knowledge does not permit us wholly to prove or wholly to disprove either of these theories; but such evidence as we possess is in favor, and increasingly in favor of the metabolic theory. All efforts to detect in the blood or in the lymph such substance as trypsinogen, or analogous substances in the case of other glands have hitherto failed; and although such a negative argument has its weakness still it is of avail as far as it goes. On the other hand, the diminution of the protoplasm in the pancreatic cell, *pari passu*, with the increase of trypsinogen, and its subsequent renewal previous to the formation of new trypsinogen, strongly support the metabolic theory, and a number of other facts drawn from the history of various animals and vegetable cells all tend strongly in the same direction. We have further a certain amount of evidence that trypsinogen arises from an antecedent more complex than itself as it in turn is more complex than trypsin. So although clear demonstration is not as yet within our reach, we may with considerable confidence conclude that trypsinogen and other like products of secreting cells arise from a breaking down of the cell substance, are manufactured by the protoplasm of the cell out of itself.

We are thus led to the conception that the specific material of a secretion such as the trypsin of pancreatic juice comes from the protoplasm of the cell, through a number of intermediate substances, or mesostates, as they are called; that is to say the complex protoplasm breaks down into a whole series of substance of decreasing complexity, the last term of which is the specific substance of the secretion. Now, the protoplasm is undoubtedly formed at the expense of the material or pabulum brought to it from the blood through the medium of the lymph; the pabulum becomes protoplasm. Here, also, two views are open to us. On the one hand, we may suppose that the cause pabulum is at once by a magic stroke, as it were, built up into the living protoplasm. On the other hand, we may suppose that the pabulum reaches the stage of protoplasm through a series of substances of increasing complexity and instability, the last stage being that which we call protoplasm. And here, too, no absolute decision between the two views is possible, but such evidence as we do possess is in favor and increasingly in favor of the latter view.

So far we have spoken of the secreting cell, but we have evidence that in the activity of a muscle a similar series of events take place reduced to theoretical simplicity, the unit, a number of which go to form a muscle, is a protoplasmic cell, undergoing like the secreting cell a continual metabolism, with a change in the results of that metabolism at the moment of functional activity. Put in a bold way, the main difference between secreting cell and a muscle cell, or elementary muscle fibre as it is often called, is that in the former the products of the metobolism constitute the main object of the cell's activity a change of form being of subordinate importance, whereas in the latter the change of form an increase of one axis at the expense of another, a shortening with corresponding thickening is the important fact, the products of the metabolism which thus gives rise to the change of form being of secondary value.

Now, we have evidence which, as in the case of the secreting cell, though not demonstrative, is weighty and of daily increasing weight, that the change of form, the contraction of a muscle is due to a sudden metabolism to an explosive decomposition of what may be called "contractile substance," a substance which appears to be used up in the act of contraction, and the consumption of which leads with other events to the exhaustion of a muscle after prolonged exertion. We know as a matter of fact that when a muscle contracts there is an evolution of a considerable quantity of carbonic acid, and a chemical change of such a kind that the muscles become acid. This carbonic acid must have some antecedent, and the acidity must have some cause. It is, of course, possible that the protoplasm itself explodes and is the immediate parent of the carbonic acid and the direct source of the energy set free in the contraction; but evidence analogous to that brought forward in relation to the secreting cell leads to the conclusion that this is not so, but that the explosion takes place in, and that the energy is derived from a specific contractile substance. And there is further evidence that this hypothetical substance to which the name of "inogen" has been provisionally given, is, like its analogue in the secreting cell, a *katastate*. So, that the contracting activity of a muscular fibre and the secreting activity of a gland cell may be compared with each other, in so far as in each case the activity is essentially a decomposition or explosion, more or less rapid, of a katastate, the inogen in the one instance, the trypsiogen or some other body in the other instance, with the setting free of energy which, in the case of the secreting cell, leaves the substance wholly as heat, but in the case of the muscle partly as movement, the activity being followed in each case by the discharge from the fibre or cell of the products, or some of the products, of this discomposition.

We may for a moment turn aside to point out that this innate difference or protoplasm serves to explain the conclusions to which modern investigation into the physiology of nutrition seem to be leading. So long as we speak of muscle or flesh as one thing the step from the flesh of mutton which we eat to the flesh of our body, which the mutton, when eaten, becomes, or may become, does not seem very far; and the older physiologists very naturally assumed that the flesh of the meal was directly without great effort and without great change, as far as mere chemical composition is concerned, transformed into the muscle of the eater. The researches, however, of modern times go to show that the substance taken as food under-

go many changes and suffer profound disruption
before they actually become part and parcel of the
living body, and, conversely, that the constructive
powers of the animal body were grossly under-
rated by earlier investigators. If one were to put
forward the thesis that the proteid of a meal becomes reduced almost to its elements before it undergoes synthesis into the superficially similar proteid of muscle, the energy set free in the destruc-
tion being utilized in the subsequent work of construction, he might appeal with confidence to modern results as supporting him rather than opposing
him in his views. It would almost seem as if the
qualities of each particle of living protoplasm were
of such an individual character that it had to be
built up afresh from almost the very beginning;
hence, the immense construction which inquiry
shows more and more clearly every day to be continually going on as well in the animal as in the
vegetable body.

Taking into consideration all the fine touches
which make up the characters of an individual organism, and remembering that these are the outcome of the different properties or activities of the
several constituent tissues of the body, working
through delicately balanced complicated machinery, bearing in mind the far-reaching phenomena
of heredity by which the gross traits and often the
minute tricks of the parents' body are reproduced

in the offspring, if there be any truth at all in the view which we have urged tracing the activities of the organism to the constitution of its protoplasm, this must be manifold indeed. The problems of physiology in the future are largely concerned in arriving, by experiment and inference, by the mind's eye, and not by the body's eye alone, assisted, as that may be, by lenses yet to be introduced, at a knowledge of the molecular construction of this protein protoplasm of the laws according to which it is built up, and the laws according to which it breaks down, for these laws when ascertained will clear up the mysteries of the protein work which the protoplasm does.

And here we may venture to introduce a word of caution. We have, in speaking of protoplasm, used the words "construction," "composition," "decomposition," and the like, as if protoplasm were a chemical substance. And it is a chemical substance in the sense that it arises out of the union or coincidence of certain factors which can be resolved into what the chemists call "elements," and can be at any time by appropriate means broken up into the same factor, and, indeed, into chemical elements.

This is not the place to enter into a discussion upon the nature of so-called chemical substances, or, what is the same thing, a discussion concerning the nature of matter; but we may venture to assert that the more these molecular problems of physiology, with which we are now dealing, are studied the stronger becomes the conviction that the consideration of what we call "structure" and "composition" must, in harmony with the modern teachings of physics, be approached under the dominant conception of modes of motion. The physicists have been led to consider the qualities of things as expressions of internal movements; even more imperative does it seem to us that the biologists should regard the qualities (including structure and composition) of protoplasm as in like manner the expression of internal movements. He may speak of protoplasm as a complex substance, but we must strive to realize that what he means by that is a complex whirl, an intricate dance, of which, what he calls chemical composition, histological structure, and gross configuration are, so to speak, the figures; to him the renewal of protoplasm is but the continuance of the dance, its functions and actions the transference of figures. In so obscure a subject it is difficult to speak otherwise than by parables, and we may call to mind how easy it is to realize the comparison of the whole body of a man to a fountain of water, as the figure of the fountain remains the same though fresh water is continually rising and falling, so the body seems the same though the fresh food is always replacing the old man, which, in turn, is always falling back to dust. And the conception which we are urging now is one which carries an analgous idea unto the study of all the molecular phenomena of the body. We must not pursue the subject any further here, but we felt it necessary to introduce the caution concerning the word "substance," and we may repeat the assertion that it seems to us necessary for a satisfactory study of the problems of which we have been dwelling for the last few pages, to keep clearly before the mind the conception that the phenomena in question are the result not of properties of kinds of matter in the vulgar sense of these words, but of kinds of motions.

In the above brief sketch we have dealt chiefly with such well known physiological actions as secretion, muscular contractions, and nervous impulses. But we must not hide from ourselves the fact that these grosser activities do not comprise the whole life of the tissues. Even in simple tissues, and more especially in the highly developed nervous tissues, there are finer actions which the conception outlined above, wholly fails to cover.

Two sets of vital phenomena have hitherto baffled inquirers, the phenomena of spontaneous activity, rhythmic or other, and the phenomena of "inhibition." All attempts to explain what actually takes place in the inner working of the tissues concerned when impulses passing down the pneumogastric nerve stop the heart from beating, or, in the many other analogous instances of the arrest of activity through activity, have signally failed; the superficial resemblance to the physical "interference of waves," breaks down upon examination, as, indeed, do all other hypothesis which have as yet been brought forward. And we are wholly in the dark as to why one piece of protoplasm or muscular fibre or nervous tissue remains quiescent till stirred by some stimulus, while another piece explodes into activity at rythmic intervals. We may frame analogies and may liken phenomena to those of a constant force rythmically overcoming a constant resistance, but such analogies bring us very little nearer to understanding what the molecules of the part are doing at and between the repeated moments of activity.

Further, if the ingenious speculation of Herieng, that specific color sensations are due to the relation of assimilation (anabolism) to dissimilation (katabolism) of protoplasmic visual substances in the retina or in the brain, should finally pass from the condition of speculation to that of demonstrated truth, we should be brought face to face with the fact that the mere act of building up or the mere act of breaking down affects the condition of protoplasm in other ways than the one which we have hitherto considered, viz: that the building up provides energy to be set free, and the breaking down lets the energy forth. In Hering's conception the mere condition of the protoplasm, whether it is largely built up or largely broken down, produces effects which result in a particular state of consciousness. Now, whatever views we may take of consciousness we must suppose that an affection of consciousness is dependent on a change in some material. But in the case of color sensations that material cannot be the visual substance itself, but some other substance. That is to say, according to Hering's views, the mere condition of the visual substance as distinct from a change in that condition determines the change in the other substance, which is the basis of consciousness. So that if Hering's conception be a true one, (and the arguments in favor of it, if not wholly conclusive, are at least serious), we are led to entertain the idea that, in addition to the rough propagation of explosive decompositions, there are continually passing from protoplasm to protoplasm delicate touches compared with which the nervous impulses which with such difficulty the galvanometer makes known to us are gross and coarse shocks. And it is at least possible, if not probable, (indeed present investigations seem rapidly tending in this direction), that an extension of Hering's view with such modifications as future inquiry may render necessary to other processes than visual sensation, more especially to the inner working of the central nervous system, may not only carry us a long way on towards understanding inhibition and spontaneous activity but may lay the foundation of a new molecular physiology. This, however, is speculative and dangerous ground. But it seemed desirable to touch upon it since it illustrates a possible or probable new departure. What we have said of it and of the more managable molecular problems of physiology will perhaps show that vast and intricate as is the maze before the physiologist today, he has in his hand a clew which promises at least to lead him far on through it.

Space forbids our entering upon a discussion concerning the methods of physiology; but accepting the truth of the preceding discussion as to the nature of physiological problems, the means of solving these problems speak for themselves.

From the earliest times the methods of physiological inquiry have belonged to one of two catagories—they have been anatomical or experimental. And the same distinction holds good today, though both methods are often joined together in one inquiry, and, indeed, at times may be said to merge the one into the other. By the anatomical method the observer ascertains the gross outlines, the minute structure, and, if necessary, the physical characters and the chemical composition of an organism, or part of an organism; and by comparison of these with those of different organism, or of the same organism placed by nature, that is, not by himself in different circumstances, he draws conclusions as to the actions taking place in it while it was alive. In early times the comparison or gross structures gave important results, but they have now been to a great extent exhausted; and the most valuable conclusions reached at the present day by the anatomical method are those arrived at by histological investigation of minute structures and by chemical analysis. The marks of this method are that on the one hand it deals for the most part with things which are no longer alive, and hence must necessarily fail to make touch with the inner workings of which we have spoken above; and, on the other hand, in its comparison of organism under different conditions it has to wait till Providence brings about what it requires, and has to be satisfied with such differences as the chapter of accidents provides. In the experimental method the observer places the organism, or part of organism, under conditions of his own choosing and applies to the organism under those conditions the same analysis as in the former methods. He ascertains changes in the gross features, minute structure, physical characters, and chemical compositions as before. So that in reality the two methods are in part identical and differ chiefly by the fact that in the latter the observer chooses the conditions in which to place the organism. But an important corollary follows, viz: that by choosing his own condition the observer is able to bring his analysis to bear on an organism or part of an organism while still alive.

The history of physiology, especially in recent times, shows that this method is the one not only of the greatest fertility but one becoming more and more essential as inquiry is pushed deeper and deeper into the more abstruce parts of physiology.

If there be any truth in the sketch given above of the modern tendencies of molecular physiology it will be clear to every mind that the experimental method alone can in the future give adequate results. It might, indeed, be urged that when molecular physics has advanced far enough the molecular problems of physiology will be interpreted by its light without recourse to experiment. It will be a long waiting till that comes. Meanwhile all the power over not only the body but what is more important, the mind or man which the physiology of the future unmistakably promises must lie unused. Nor is it simply a matter of waiting, for it is at least within the range of possibility that when the molecular problems of physiology are fairly grasped conclusions may be reached which will throw back a light on the molecular processes of inanimate masses, revealing features of what we call matter which could not be discovered by the examination of bodies which had never lived.

It would not be a hard task to give chapter and verse for the assertion that the experimental method has, especially in these later times, supplied the chief means of progress in physiology; but it would be a long task, as we may content ourselves with calling attention to what is in many respects a typical case. We referred a short time back the phenomena of "inhibition." It is not too much to say that the discovery of the inhibitory function of certain nerves marks one of the most important steps in the progress of physiology during the past half century. The mere attainment of the fact that the stimulation of a nerve might stop action instead of inducing action constituted in itself almost a revolution, and the value of that fact in helping us on the one hand to unravel the tangled puzzle of physiological action and reaction, and on the other hand, to push our inquiries into the still more difficult problems of molecular changes, has proved immense. One cannot at the present time take up a physiological memoir covering any large extent of ground without finding some use made of inhibitory processes for the purpose of explaining physiological phenomena.

Now, however skillfully we may read older statements between the lines, no scientific, that is, no exact knowledge of inhibition was possessed by any physiologist until Weber, by a direct experiment on a living animal, discovered the inhibitory influence of the pneumogastric nerve over the beating of the heart. It was, of course, previously known that under certain circumstances the beating of the heart might be stopped; but all ideas as to how the stoppage was or might be brought about were vague and uncertain before Weber made his experiment. That experiment gave the clew to an exact knowledge, and it is difficult if not impossible to see how the clew could have been gained otherwise than by experiment; other experiments have enabled us to follow up the clew so that it may with justice be said that all that part of the recent progress of physiology which is due to the introduction of a knowledge of inhibitory processes is the direct result of the experimental method. But the story of our knowledge of inhibition is only one of the innumerable instances of the value of this method. In almost every department of physiology an experiment or a series of experiments has proved a turning point at which vague nebulous fancies were exchanged for clear decided knowledge or a starting point for the introduction of wholly new and startling ideas. And we may venture to repeat that not only must the experimental method be continued, but the progress of physiology will chiefly depend on the increase application of that method. The more involved and abstruе the problems become the more necessary does it also become that the inquirer should be able to choose his own conditions for the observations he desires to make. Happily, the experimental method itself brings with it in the course of its own development the power of removing the only valid objection to physiological experiments, viz: that in certain cases they involve pain and suffering. For in nearly all experiments pain and suffering are disturbing elements. These disturbing elements the present imperfect methods are often unable to overcome; but their removal will become a more and more pressing necessity in the interests of the experiments themselves, as the science becomes more exact and exacting, and will also become a more and more easy task as the progress of the science makes the investigator more and more master of the organism. In the physiology of the future pain and suffering will be admissible in an experiment only when pain and suffering are themselves the object of inquiry.

And such an inquiry will of necessity take a subjective rather than an objective form.

CHAPTER III.

TUBERCULOSIS BACILLUS are slender rods usually in pairs; not motile spores not definitely determined; facultatively *anærobic*.

Habitat in all organs and secretions of tubercular persons its chief characteristics are pathogenic, it is facultative *abærolic;* in order that the bacilli be active they must be excluded from oxygen as soon as sputa is evacuated by expectoration, there is no life or action whatever, and in order to propagate them it is necessary by culture to add serum or potatoes to sput which contains tuberculosis bacilli and encase it in air tight receptical and maintain 37° c.

Tuberculosis bacilli are in spores, hence the resistance of spores because of the very tenacious envelope the spore is not easily influenced by external measure, it is said to be the most resisting object of the organic world, chemical and physical agents that easily destroy other life have very little effect upon it, many spores require a temperature of 140° c. dry heat for several hours to destroy

140°c. dry heat for several hours to destroy them; the spores of a variety of potato bacillus can withstand the application of steam at 100°c. for four hours.

The bacilla of tuberculosis will not be impaired nor injured by boiling in nitric acid for four hours 212F. or 100°c. after process of boiling are as visible and numerous upon microscopic test, and can be developed by culture in size and number, hence to treat by inhilation it would be impossible to inhale a gas that would attack the bacilli as resistance of tissue in lungs would not be able to withstand the strain, as we know tuberculosis bacilli are *anærobic* and that oxygen is destructive to them, the one and only way to completely remove them from the system is by increasing the oxygen in the body and that can only be accomplished by restoring the lacking element in the muscular system and improving digestion which will actually follow when the muscles are strengthened.

In this work you will note list of Bacteria, Pathogenic and non-Pathogenic, and you will also note that the lungs are bacillicidal, and if sufficiently strengthened, will destroy and expel the tubercular baccilli as well as all other bacteria, as all vegetable matter is continually filling the air with bacteria which causes fever and sickness, some will contract the sickness and others won't; it is termed contagious; others will come in contract, and, in fact, care and attend the afflicted, and experience no inconvenience. How so? First, the party that contracted the disease from the afflicted one was not in good spirits, in other words, was ailing from some stomach or nervous trouble, while the immune, as we may say, was in good condition, all organs being active, and especially the stomach.

CHAPTER IV.

ESSENTIALS OF BACTERIOLOGY.

GENERAL CONSIDERATIONS.

BACTERIA.

BACTERIA (*Baxrnpov*, little staff,) is a name given to a group of the lowest form of plants, very closely following the *algæ*. They were called Fission-Fungi or Schizomycetes, (*oxica*, to cleave; *uoxns*, fungus,) because it was thought that, as the fungi, they lived without the *chlorophyll*. The word fission was supplied to distinguish them from moulds and yeasts; it denoting the manner of reproduction. Since several bacteria have been found to possess *chlorophyll*, and as a great many increase in other ways than by simple fission, the name of Schizomycetes can no longer be applied, though the word Bacteria leaves much to be desired.

Classification. Ferdinand Cohn, in the middle of the present century, was the first to demonstrate bacteria to be of vegetable origin, they being placed previous to that among the *infusoria*. He arranged them according to their form under four divisions.

Cohn's System.
I. *Spherobacteria*, (globules),
II. *Microbatceria*, (short rods),
III. *Desmobacteria*, (long rods),
IV. *Spirobacteria*, (spirals),

as expressed at the present time, Micrococcus, Baccilus, and Spirillum. This classification is very superficial, but because a better one has not been found it is most in use today.

DeBary's System. DeBary divides bacteria into two groups, those arising from or giving rise to endospores and those developed from arthrospores. This division has a more scientific value than the first.

Structure. Bacteria are cells; they appear as round or cylindrical, of an average diameter or transverse section of 0.001mm, (1 micromillimeter), written 1u. The cell, as other plant cells, is composed of a membranous cell wall and cell contents; "cell nuclei" have not yet been observed, but the latest researches point to their presence.

Cell Wall. The cell wall is composed of plant cellulose, which can be demonstrated in some cases by the tests for cellulose. The membrane is firm and can be brought plainly into view by the action of iodine upon the cell contents which contracts them.

Cell Contents. The contents of the cell consist mainly of protoplasm usually homogeneous, but in some varieties finely granular, or holding pigment, chlorophyll, granulose, and sulphur in its structure.

It is composed chiefly of mycoprotein.

Gelatinous Membrane. The outer layer of the cell membrane can absorb water and become glatinoid, forming either a little envelope or capsule around the bacterium or preventing the separation of the newly branched germs, forming chains and bunches as strepto and staphylo-cocci. Long filaments are also formed.

Zoogloea. When this gelatinous membrane is very thick, irregular masses of bacteria will be formed, the whole growth being in one jelly-like lump. This is termed a zoogloea (*zoow*, animal; *aoug*, glue).

Locomotion. Many bacteria possess the faculty of self-movement, carrying themselves in all manner of ways across the micropscopic field, some very quickly, others leisurely.

Vibratory Movements. Some bacteria vibrate in themselves, appearing to move, but they do not change their place; these movements are denoted as molecular or Brownian.

Flagella. Little threads or lashes are found attached to many of the motile bacteria, either at the poles or along the sides, sometimes only one, and on some several, forming a tuft.

These flagella are in constant motion, and can probably be considered as the organs of locomotion; they have not yet been discovered upon all the motile bacteria, owing no doubt to our imperfect methods of observation. They can be stained and have been photographed.

Reproduction. Bacteria multiply either through simple division or through fructification by means of small round or oval bodies called spores, from *spora* (seed). In the first case division, the cell elongates, and at one portion, usually the middle, the cell wall indents itself gradually, forming a septum, and dividing the cell into two equal parts, just as occurs in the higher plant and animal cells.

Spore Formations. Two forms of sporulation: Endosporous and Arthrosporous. First, a small granule developes in the protoplasm of a bacterium, this increases in size, or several little granules coalesce to form an elongate, highly refractive, clearly defined object, rapidly attaining its real size, and this is the spore. The remainder of the cell contents has now disappeared, leaving the spore in a dark, very resistant membrane or capsule, and beyond this the weak cell wall. The cell wall dissolves gradually or stretches and allows the spore to be set free.

Each bacterium gives rise to but one spore. It may be at either end or in the middle. Some rods take on a peculiar shape at the side of the spore, making the rod look like a drum-stick or spindle—*clostridium*.

Spore Contents. What the real contents of spores are is not known. In the mother cell at the site of the spore little granules have been found which stain differently from the rest of the cell, and these are supposed to be the beginnings, the sporogenic bodies. The most important part of the spore is its capsule; to this it owes its resisting properties. It consists of two separate layers, a thin membrane around the cell and a firm outer gelatinous envelope.

Germination. When brought into favorable conditions the spore begins to lose its shining appearance, the outer firm membrane begins to swell, and it now assumes the shape and size of the cell from which it sprang, the capsule having burst, so as to allow the young bacillus to be set free.

Requisites for Spore Formation. It was formerly thought that when the substratum could no longer maintain it, or had become infiltrated with detrimental products, the bacterium cell produced spores, or rather turned itself into a spore to escape annihilation; but we know that only when the conditions are the most favorable to the well being of the cell, does it produce fruit, just as with every other type of plant or animal life, a certain amount of oxygen and heat being necessary for good spore formation.

Asporogenic Bacteria. Bacteria can be so damaged that they will remain sterile, not produce any spores. This condition can be temporary only, or permanent.

Arthrosporous. All the above remarks relate to Endospores, spores that arise within the cells.

In the other group, called Arthrospores, individual members of a colony or aggregation leave the same, and become the originators of new colonies, thus assuming the character of spores.

The Micrococci furnish examples of this form.

Some authorities have denied the existence of the arthrosporous formation.

Resistance of Spores. Because of the very tenacious envelope the spore is not easily influenced by external measures. It is said to be the most resisting object of the organic world.

Chemical and physical agents that easily desstroy other life have very little effect upon it.

Many spores require a temperature of 140°c. dry heat for several hours to destroy them. The spores of a variety of potato bacillus (bacillus mesentericus) can withstand the application of steam at 100°c. for four hours.

ORIGIN OF BACTERIA AND THEIR DISTRIBUTION.

As Pasteur has shown, all bacteria develop from pre-existing bacteria, or the spores of the same. They cannot, do not arise *de novo*.

Their wide and almost universal diffusion is due to the minuteness of the cells and the few requirements of their existence.

Very few places are free from germs; the air on the high seas, and on the mountain tops, is said to be free from bacteria, but it is questionable.

One kind of bacterium will not produce another kind.

A bacillus does not arise from a micrococcus or the typhoid fever bacillus produce the bacillus of tetanus.

This subject has been long and well discussed, and it would take many pages to state the pros and cons, therefore this positive statement is made, it being the position now held by the principal authorities.

Saprophytes and Parasites. (*Saprophytes*, putrid plant; Parasites, aside of food.) Those bacteria which live on the dead remains of organic life are known as Saprophytic Bacteria, and those which choose the living bodies of their fellow creatures for their habitat are called Parisitic Bacteria. Some, however, develop equally well as saprophytes and parasites. They are called Facultative Parasites.

Conditions of Life and Growth of Bacteria. Influence of temperature. In general a temperature ranging from 10°c. to 40°c. is necessary to their life and growth.

Saprophytes take the lower temperatures; parasites, the temperature more approaching the animal heat of the warm-blooded. Some forms require a nearly constant heat, growing within very small limits, as the Bacillus of Tuberculosis.

Some forms can be arrested in their development by a warmer or colder temperature, and then restored to activity by a return to the natural heat.

A few varieties exist only at freezing point of water; and others again that will not live under a temperature of 60°c.

For the majority of Bacteria a temperature of 60°c. is destructive and several times freezing and thrawing very fatal.

Influence of Oxygen.—Two varieties of bacteria in relation to oxygen. The one ærobic, growing in air; the other anærobic, living without air.

Obligate ærobins; those which exist only when oxygen is present.

Facultative ærobins; those that live best when oxygen is present, but can live without it.

Obligate or true anærobins; those which can not exist where oxygen is.

Facultative anærobins; those which exist better where there is no oxygen but can live in its presence.

Some derive the oxygen which they require out of their nutriment, so that a bacterium may be ærobic and yet not require the presence of free oxygen.

Ærobins may consume the free oxygen of a regin and thus allow the anærobins to develop. By improved methods of culture many varieties of anærobins have been discovered.

Influence of Light.—Sunlight is very destructive to bacteria. A few hours exposure to the sun has been fatal to anthrax bacilli, and the cultures of bacillus tuberculosis have been killed by a few days' standing in daylight.

Vital Actions of Microbes. Bacteria feeding upon organic compounds produce chemical changes in them, not only by the withdrawal of certain elements but also by the exertion of these elements changed by digestion. Sometimes such changes are destructive to themselves, as when lactic and butyric acids are formed in the media.

Oxidation and reduction are carried on by some bacteria. Ammonia, hydrogensulphide, and trimethylamin are a few of the chemical products produced by bacteria.

Ptomaines. Brieger found a number of complex alkaloids, closely resembling those found in ordinary plants, and which he named Ptomaines (*corpse*) because obtained from putrefying objects.

Fermentation. This form of " splitting up — fermentation, as it is called—is due to the direct action of vegetable organism. Many bacteria have the power of ferments.

Putrefaction. When fermentation is accompanied by development of offensive gasses, a decomposition occurs, which is called putrefaction; and this, in organic substance, is due entirely to bacteria.

Liquefaction of Solid Gelatine. Some varieties of bacteria digest the nutrient gelatine, and so dissolve it; others execrete a ferment which liquifies the gelatine.

Producers of Disease. Various pathological processes are caused by bacteria, the name given to such diseases being infectious diseases and the germs themselves called disease-producing pathogenic bacteria. Those which do not form any pathological process are called non-pathogenic bacteria.

Pigmentation. Some bacteria are endowed with the property of forming pigments either in themselves, or producing a chromogenic body which, when set free, gives rise to the pigment. In some cases the pigments have been isolated and many of the properties of the aniline dyes discovered in them.

Phosphoresence. Many bacteria have the power to form light giving to various objects which they inhabit a characteristic glow or phosphoresence.

Fluorescence. An iridescence, or play of colors, develops in some of the bacterial cultures.

Gas Formation. Many bacteria, anærobic ones especially, produce gases, noxious and odorless; in the culture media the bubbles which arise soon displace the media.

Odors. Some germs form odors characteristic of them; some sweet, aromatic ones, and other ones very foul, disagreeable smells; some give a sour or ransid exhalation.

Effect of Age. With age bacteria lose their strength and die. Bacteria thus carry on all the functions of higher organized life; they breathe, eat, digest, execrete and multiply; and they are very busy workers.

CHAPTER V.

SCROFULA.

DEFINITION.—A constitutional disease, marked by abnormal nutrition and production of cells, resulting either in the deposits of tubercle or in specific forms of inflammation or ulceration. It may be associated with Tuberculosis or it may occur without.

SCROFULA WITH TUBERCLE.—It is at present uncertain whether Scrofula and Tuberculosis are different diseases or not, but it is highly probable that the disease of the blood which leads to the growth of tubercles and that which gives the specific character of scrofulous affections are identical.

Tubercles are about as large as millet seeds, and are of two varieties, the grey and yellow; the former is semi-transparent and somewhat firm; the latter of a dull, yellow color, and of a cheesy consistence. The yellow has in it far greater elements of danger; softening takes place earlier, and it has a greater tendency to aggregate in masses. Frequently the two varieties are mixed; but as cases advance towards a fatal termination the yellow appears to gain the ascendency. Many pathologists are of the opinion that the yellow is simply the grey tubercle in a state of caseous degeneration and that an uncertain interval elapses before the degeneration occurs.

Tubercles are usually produced slowly and painlessly during some period of defective health, and after remaining latent for an indefinite time they waste, or calcify, if the general health improves, or soften and cause abscesses and other destructive changes, if the health deterioates. Unlike cancer, tubercle has no elements of reproduction.

The practical conclusions of Laennec, Clark, Bennett, Pollock, and other scientific observers are that if the further growth of tubercle can be arrested, those already existing may diminish in size, become absorbed, and the parts cicatrize; or they may remain dormant without exciting any symptoms, after undergoing a process called certification, in which the animal portion is absorbed, the earthly only remaining. Frequently, however, from defective hygienic conditions, or other cause, tubercles undergo a succession of changes; they first become soft in the center, that part being the oldest and most removed from living influences; then, like foreign bodies, they excite inflammation, suppuration, and ulcertion in the neighboring tissue. The groups often continue to enlarge till several groups communicate and form a vomica; this bursts, and when the lungs are the organs involved its contents are discharged into an adjacent bronchial tube, and the matter is conveyed into the windpipe, and thence to the mouth, to be evacuated. Unless the disease be arrested other abscesses form and unite till the lung substance is so diminished in volume, and its continuity so completely destroyed as to be incompatible with life, and the patient dies of exhaustion. In other cases, under the treatment, the tubercular matter, with the inflammatory products it excited, are removed by expectoration or absorption, the tissue around the cavity contract and obliterate it, and so the disease is cured.

The parts most commonly affected by tubercle are the lungs, the brain and its membrane, the liver, the intestines, the pericardium, and the peritoneum.

(*b*) Scrofula without Tubercle is usually manifested by various local lesions, the most common of which is induration and enlargement of the subcataneous glands of the neck, below the jaws, in the axillae, or groins, and less frequently in other parts of the body. These swellings are at first soft, painless, movable; afterwards they may enlarge, become painful, inflame and eventually suppurate, forming scrofulous ulcers. They occur very frequently during childhood, and are excited into activity by Cold, Measles, Scarlatina, Whooping Cough, etc., and either remain for a long time inoperative, or proceed to inflammation and suppuration. Not that all enlargements of the lymphatic vessels and glands are due to scrofula; they may arise from temporary causes, and their character as such is readily determined by the history and symptoms they present.

CAUSES.—The most important predisposing cause is hereditary tendency. But the following may be both predisposing and exciting causes, and their power in the production of struma can hardly be overstated.

Want of pure air, consequent on the imperfect ventilation of sitting and sleeping rooms, is a frequent and potent exciting cause of tubercular disease, as indeed might be inferred from the physiological evidence of the extreme importance of a proper aeration of the blood. Persons breathing for a considerable period, air which has been rendered impure by respiration, soon become pale, partially lose their appetite and gradual decline in strength and spirits.

Unhealthy occupations rank among the predisposing causes of scrofulous disease. But occupations are only injurious to health incidentally and the chief circumstances which render them so are mostly preventable and are briefly the following. Deficiency of sunlight and pure air, the inhalation of mechanical or poisonous substances, too prolonged hours of work, a bad posture of the body during labor, and the intemperance, and consequent poverty of those engaged in them. Outdoor occupations are much less likely to produce scrofulous or tuberculous disease than those practiced indoors.

A deficient supply or an improper quality of food may serve as an exciting cause, although probably to a less extent than causes already pointed out.

CHAPTER VI.

TREATMENT.—The perfection of the treatment of scrofula and tubercle, as, indeed, of disease in general, lies in its adaption to individual cases. The stock whence the patient has sprung, the circumstances of birth and early life, education and general habits, the influence of soil and climate, the disease passed through the tendency to disease of the body generally, and of organs and tissues in particular, these are but illustrations of the points that have to be brought under consideration before a course of treatment can be prudently decided upon. The treatment is generally tedious often requiring to be continued for months, or even years in extreme cases.

First. The remedies are well adapted to those constitutions in which the digestion and assimilation of food does not lead to the formation of good blood and healthy tissue. There is an impoverished, or on the other hand, a stout, soft, and pale appearance, notwithstanding that a sufficient supply of good food is partaken of. It is indicated in the cases of enlarged and hard abdomen, so frequently met with in children with a tuberculous tendency. Other indications for this remedy are a want of firmness of the bones, slow or difficult dentition, scrofulous swellings, extreme sensitiveness to cold and damp.

Second. The Remedies are beneficial for the treatment of unhealthy skin; scrofulous ophthalmia of children; humid eruptions behind, or purient discharge from the ears; swelling of the axillulry glands, tonsils, nose or upper lip; swelling of the upper knee, hip or other joints; defective nutrition; colicky pains, mucus discharges, etc.

Also for frequently and easily disordered lungs, with a short dry cough, pain or soreness of the chest, shortness of breath, tendency to diarrhœa or prespiration, and general feebleness of constitution.

Third. It is of great value to the anœmic, impoverish, and cachectic condition so common in scrofula and tuberculosis, arising from imperfect assimilation of food.

Also for scrofulous ulcers with callous edges, fistulous ulcers, scale head, otorrhœa; scrofulous affections of the bones. It may follow calc., especially in diseases of the bones.

Fourth. Glandular inflammation with much swelling, redness, and the pains worse at night in bed, particularly when the glands of the neck are swollen and painful, and there are strumous affections of the eyes; copious saliva, disagreeable taste and frequent and unhealthy-looking stools. Also females with menstrual irregularities, corrosive leucorrhœa, indurations of the uterus, unclear skin, etc.

Fifth. Enlargement of the glands; scrofulous inflammation of the knee, rough dry skin, enlarged mesenteric glands, and tender abdomen; amaciated appearance, with hectic. A chronic diarrhœa, premonitory of consumption of the bowels, is well met by this remedy.

Sixth. Indigestion with flatulence, heartburn, acid eructations, and constipation or irregular action of the bowels. It is especially indicated in patients of dark compexion, sallow skin, or sedentary habits, or who suffer much from mental fatigue or anxiety.

Seventh. In addition to the indications before pointed out, this remedy is useful in obstinate acid eructations, and when a debilitating relaxation of the bowels is present.

Eighth. Faulty action of the liver, shown in yellowish skin and conjunctive, mental depression, anorexia, etc.

ACCESSORY MEANS.—These are of the greatest importance, for medicine will be of little use unless hygienic rules are strictly adhered to.

AIR.—Pure, fresh air is required night and day. Scrofulous residents are rarely found near the seaside. The larger the sleeping rooms the better; the fireplace should be open; the temperature about 55 degrees.

EXERCISE.—Moderate exercise in the open air is most essential; and in carrying out this suggestion the patient should endeavor to take exercise with the mind agreeably occupied, rather than following it as an irksome task. Moderate gymnastic exercise is beneficial, but profuse prespiration should be avoided.

FOOD.—The food of scrofulous patients should always be of the most nutritious character, light and digestible. Beef, mutton, venison, and fowls are the best kind of animal food; to these should be added preparations of eggs and milk, a due quantity of bread, mealy potatoes, rice, and other farinaceous principals as more suited to this class of patients than watery and succulent vegetables.

COD LIVER OIL, as a supplemental article of diet, is an agent possessing such remarkable and well known properties of arresting general or local emaciation as not to require further recommendation here. It may be given in almost any case in which a patient is losing flesh, in teaspoonful doses two or three times a day, commencing even with half a teaspoonful, if it be found first to disagree.

BATHING, both in fresh and salt water, is invaluable as a means of promoting a healthy action of the skin, and of imparting tone to the whole system.

CLOTHING should be adapted to the season, and should be warm without being oppressive. The extremities especially should be kept warm. Flannel should be worn; in the winter it affords direct warmth, and in summer it tends to neutralize the effects of sudden changes of temperature. The linen should be frequently changed, always observing that it is put on perfectly dry.

PREVENTION.—The prevention of strumous disease consists not alone in the hygienic or medical treatment of the patients, but primarily in the correction of habits, and improving the health of the parents, more particular in respect to the points referred to under "Causes."

CHAPTER VII.

PULMONARY TUBERCULOSIS.

An infectious disease due to the introduction into the system of the bacilli tuberculosis discovered by Koch in 1882, it has a very wide spread, almost a universal distribution, and it is estimated that fully one-seventh of all mankind die of it; the bacilli, the essential etiologic, gains entrance into the body with the inspired air, with the food, and direct inoculation. The commonest mode of introduction is by inhalation; in consequence the respiratory tract is the most frequent seat of tuberculosis. The bacilli become disseminated in the air chiefly through the agency of the sputum of persons afflicted with pulmonary tuberculosis. The sputum of such individuals contains countless bacilli, which are held in it as long as it is moist, but are scattered through the air when the sputum becomes dry and pulverulent. When tuberculosis is acquired through food, an occurence not rare in childhood, it localizes itself primarily in the intestinal tract. The food which most often conveys the disease is milk from tuberculosis animals, more rarely tuberculous meat. Direct inoculation does not play an important role in the causation of the disease. The status of heredity as a factor in the propagation of tuberculosis is not yet fully settled. Isolated instances of apparently hereditary transmission, both in man and in animals, are recorded, and demonstrate that the disease may be inherited should hereditary tendency be prevalent in family history, it is not likely that any signs of it will be manifested should proper care be taken and avoid colds and keep up the system to highest possible degree, when the system is active it is entirely immune, and when tuberculosis bacillus is inhaled it is instantly expelled by chemical action of the lungs, but should the system be exhausted from overwork, worry, or sickness, and then subjected to tuberculosis bacilli by inhalation, the system would not be immune and would not have required chemical action to act as bacillicidal. But in the majority of cases the acquisition of tuberculosis is post-natal. There is, however, a manifest tendency of the disease to attack the offspring of tuberculos parents, which as it is not the result of hereditary transmission, must indicate the existence of a predisposition or susceptibility which is transmitted from parent to child. The lesion produced by the growth of the bacillus of tuberculosis is known as the Tubercle (miliary, or gray, or nodule). This is small, grayish, translucent nodule, from one-tenth to 2mm. in diameter, firmly imbedded in the surrounding tissues. By the coalescence of neighboring tubercles larger masses the so-called tuberculous infiltrations are produced. Histologically a typical tubercle consists of three groups of cells. the epithelioia, the giant cells, and the round or lymphoid cells. The first are oval in shape, have a vesicular nucleus, and are the result of the proliferation of the fixed connective tissue and endothelial cells; perhaps also of epithelial cells. The formation of oval cells is the first effect produced by the tubercle bacillus. The giant cell is a large multinuclear mass, usually situated in the center of the tubercle. It may be the product of repeated muclear multiplication in a single cell, without division of the cell protoplasm, or the result of the coalescence of several adjacent cells. The round cells are leukocytes that have emigrated from the blood vessels, and they may be so numerous as to conceal the other cells (Lymphoid tubercle). The bacilli are found in the giant cells between and in the epithelioia cells, and in later stages in the round cells. New blood vessels are not formed in the tubercle.

The tendency of the tuberculous formation is to undergo a peculiar form of coagulation known as cheesy necrosis. This gives rise to a structureless, yellowish-white mass, which microscopically shows an almost total absence of nuclei in the central area, while in the periphery nuclei both normal and in various stages of degeneration are found. The necrotic tissue does not as a rule take any stain. For this degeneration two factors are responsible—the absence of blood vessels and the actions of peculiar poisons elaborated by the bacillus. The breaking down of tuberculous areas in the interior of the organs give rise to cavities which may be seen in muscles, bones, brain, lmphatic glands and elsewhere, but are most pronounced in the lungs, where they may attain a very large size.

I will now endeavor to explain the condition of the system that is favorable to the propagation of tuberculosis. In no case can the bacillus be effective if the organs are active and performing their respective functions, and in no case is the system safe from the ravages of the tubercular diseases if debilitated. Pulmonary tuberculosis can and does attack persons who have had no hereditary tendency in their family history, but was superinduced by overwork, worry, and neglected colds, reducing their vitality to such extent that the muscular action of the lungs are impaired.

Tuberculosis in no case can gain any perceptible headway until such time as the nervous system is affected, and in no case can any symptoms be apparent until such time that digestion and assimilation is impaired to such extent that the supply of blood is not equal to the demand and in consequence of the muscular weakness.

CHAPTER VIII.

THEREFORE

PULMONARY TUBERCULOSIS

is caused from vital force being reduced, thereby affecting the respiratory organ; it being generally understood that when the system is run down that there is lack of red corpuscles in the blood; the cause of the deficient red corpuscles is a lack of oxygen in the blood, principally caused by the lungs being somewhat congested, and when such is the case then the lungs are unable to exhale the carbonic acid gas, the carbonic case of itself will destroy the hamoglobin off the blood, which constitutes more than ninety per cent. of the bulk of the corpuscles of the blood.

It must be, therefore, evident that the chief part of oxygen is contained in the corpuscles, and not in a state of simple solution, the chief solid constituent of the colored corpuscles is hamoglobin, which constitute more than ninety per cent. of their bulk.

This body has a very marked affinity for oxygen, absorbing it to a very definite extent, under favorable circumstances, and giving it up when subjected to the actions of reducing agents, or to a sufficiently low oxygen pressure, from these facts it is inferred that oxygen of the blood is combined with hamoglobin and not simply dissolved, but inasmuch as it is comparatively easy to cause the hamoglobin to give up its oxygen, it is believed that the oxygen is but loosely combined with the substance.

The respiratory mechanism respiration consists of the alternate expansion and contraction of the thorax by means of which air is drawn into or expelled from the lungs, the acts are called inspiration expiration, respectively, for the inspiration of the air into the lungs it is evident that all that is necessary is such a movement of the side walls or floor of the chest, or both, that the capacity of the interior shall be enlarged by such increase of capacity, there will be of course a diminution of pressure of the air in the lungs, and a fresh quantity will enter through the larnyx trachea to equalize the pressure on the inside and outside of the chest for the inspiration of air, on the other hand is also evident that by an opposite movement which shall diminish the capacity of the chest the pressure in the interior will increase and air will be expelled until the pressure within and without the chest are again equal.

In both cases the air passes through the trachea and larynx whether in entering or leaving the lungs; there being no other communication with the exterior of the lungs; and the lungs for the same reason remain under all circumstances described closely in contact with the walls and floor of the chest; to speak of expansion of the chest, is to speak also of expansion of the lungs.

We will now consider the means by which the respiratory movements are affected. Inspiratory muscles, and in the laternal and autero-posterior diameters, the muscles engaged in ordinary inspiration are the diaphragm, the external intercostal, the levatores costarum, and serratus posticus superior. The vertical diameter of the chest is increased by the contraction and consequently descent of the diaphragm the sides of the muscles descending most and the central tendon remaining comparatively unmoved, while the intercostal and other muscles, by acting at the same, prevent the diaphragm during its contraction from drawing in the sides of the chest, thereby we understand why there is not the necessary per cent. of the red corpuscles in the blood, and it being necessary to replenish them before we can hope for a cure, in order to do so we must feed the nerves and muscles and thereby strengthen the respirator mechanism.

The Clancy Discoveries which are now administered by The St. Phillip's Remedies Company is a specific having the medicinal properties to meet those necessary requirements.

First, the Remedies have power to relieve intense suffering; second, the Remedies are most efficacious in stopping the diarrhœa; third, they act like a tonic upon the mucous membrane of the stomach, and, facilitating the digestion, create an appetite, the stomach being, however, connected with higher nerve centers by means of branches of the vagua and of the splanchnic nerves through the solar plexus by the stimulant which the medicine contains the nerves are fed and vitality is restored, and the lungs are once more able to perform their function.

We maintain that our Remedies will cure ninety-eight per cent. when in first stage of consumption, and at least seventy-five per cent. when in second stage, and in third and last stage it will not cure those, but will relieve and render the tubercular bacilli innocuous, so it cannot be propagated. The medicine is a liquid, and is administered internally from three to four times daily, as the case may require. For children, proportional to age.

Patients cannot use BEER in any form; good liquors taken moderately will not be detrimental.

CHAPTER IX.

PNEUMONIA.

PNEUMONIA, or inflammation of the substance of the lungs, manifests itself in several forms which differ from each other in their nature, causes, and results, viz: (1) Acute Croupous, or Lobar Pneumonia, the most common form of the disease, in which the inflammation affects a limited area, usually a lobe or lobes of the lung, and runs a rapid course. (2). Catarrhal Pneumonia, Broncho Pneumonia, or Lobular Pneumonia, which occurs as a result of antecedent bronchitis, and is more diffuse in its distribution than the former. (3). Interstitial Pneumonia, or Cirrhosis of the Lung, a more chronic form of inflammation, which affects chiefly the frame-work of fibrous stroma of the lung and is closely allied to phthisis.

Acute Croupous, or Lobar Pneumonia. This is the disease commonly known as Inflammation of the Lungs. It derives its name from its pathological characters, which are well marked. The changes which take place in the lung are chiefly three. (1). Congestion, or engorgement, the blood vessels being distended and the lung more voluminous and heavier than normal, and of dark red color. Its air cells still contain air. (2). Red Hepatization, so called from its resemblance to liver tissue. In this stage there is poured into the air cells of the affected part an exudation consisting of amorphous fibrim, together with epithelial cells and red and white blood corpuscels, the whole forming a viscid mass which occupies not only the cells but also the finer bronchi, and which speedily coagulates, causing the lung to become firmly consolidated. In this condition the cells are entirely emptied of air, their blood vessels are pressed upon by the exudation, and the lung substance, rendered brittle, sinks in water. The appearance of a section of the lung in this stage has been likened to that of red granite. It is to the character of the exudation, consisting largely of coagulable fibrin, that the term croupous is due. (3). Gray Hepatization. In this stage the lung retains its liver-like consistence, but its color is now gray, not unlike the appearance of gray granite. This is due to the change taking place in the exudation, which undergoes solution by a process of fatty degeneration, pus formation, liquefaction, and ultimately absorption, so that in a comparatively short period the air vessels get rid of their morbid contents and resume their normal function. This is, happily, the termination of the majority of cases of croupous pneumonia, yet it occasionally happens that this favorable result is not attained, and that further changes of a retrograde kind take place in the inflamed lung in the form of suppuration and abscess or of gangrene. In such instances there usually exists some serious constitutional cause which constitutes to give this unfavorable direction to the course of the disease. Further, pneumonia may in some instances become chronic, the lung never entirely clearing up, and it may terminate in phthisis. Pneumonia may be confined to a portion or the whole of one lung, or it may be double, affecting both lungs, which is a serious and often fatal form. The bases or middle of the lungs are the parts most commonly inflamed, but the apex is sometimes the only part affected. The right lung is considerably more frequently the seat of pneumonia than the left lung.

Many points in the pathology of this form of pneumonia remain still to be cleared up. Thus there is a growing opinion that it is not a simple lung inflammation, as was formerly supposed, but that as regards its origin, progress, and termination it possesses many of the characters of a fever or of a constitutional affection. An interesting and important fact in this connection is the recent discovery by Friedlander and others of a micro-organism or bacillus in the blood and lungs, and other tissues in cases of pneumonia, which when inoculated into certain lower animals is followed by the symptoms and appearances characteristic of that disease. Still it must be confessed that such inoculation experiments carried on in rabbits, guinea pigs or mice are scarcely sufficient by themselves to settle the question of the specific and infectious nature of pneumonia as it affects the human subject, yet they are of distinct value as evidence pointing in that direction. Further, there are numerous instances on record in which this disease has appeared to spread as an epidemic in localities or in families in such a way as strongly to suggest the idea of infectiveness. Cases of this kind, however, are open to the question as to whether there may not coexist some other disease such as fever, of which the pneumonia present is but a complication. The whole subject of the pathology of pneumonia is still under investigation, and all that can in the meantime be affirmed is that it presents many features which render its phenomena unlike those of an ordinary inflammation, while on the other hand it has strong analogies to some of the specific fevers. As regards known causes, in the vast majority of instances an attack of pneumonia comes on as the result of exposure to cold as the exciting agent, while such conditions as fatigue and physical or mental depression are often traceable as powerful predisposing influences.

The symptoms of acute pneumonia are generally well marked from the beginning. The attack is usually ushered in by a rigor, (or in children, a convulsion), together with vomiting and the speedy development of the febrile condition, the temperature rising to a considerable degree—101° to 104° or more. The pulse is quickened, and there is a marked disturbance in the respiration, which is rapid, shallow and difficult, the rate being usually accelerated to some two or three times its normal amount. The lips are livid and the face has a dusky flush. Pain in the side is felt, especially should any amount of pleurisy be present, as is often the case. Cough is an early symptom. It is at first frequent and hacking, and is accompanied with a little tough colorless expectoration, which soon, however, becomes more copious and of a rusty brown color, either tenacious or frothy and liquid. Microscopically this consists mainly of ephithelium casts of the air cells, and fine bronchi, together with granular matter and blood and pus corpuscles.

The following are the chief physical signs in tne various stages of the disease: In the stage of real hepatization the affected side of the chest is seen to expand less freely than the opposite side; there is dullness on percussion and increase of the vocal fremitus, while on auscultation the breath sounds are tubular or bronchial in character; with it may be some amount of fine crepitation, in certain parts in the stage of gray hepatization the percussion note is still dull and the breathing tubular, but crepitations of coarser quality than before are also audible. These various physical signs disappear more or less rapidly during convalesence. With the progess of the inflammation the febrile symptoms and rapid breathing continue. The patient during the greater part of the disease lies on the back or on the affected side. The pulse, which at first was full, becomes small and soft owing to the interruption to the pulmonary circulation. Occasionally slight jaundice is present, due probably to a similar cause. The urine is scanty, sometimes albuminous, and its chlorides arc diminishes. In favorable cases, however severe, there generally occurs after six or eight days a distinct crises, marked by a rapid fall of the temperature, accompanied with perspiration and with copious discharge of lithates in the urine.

Although no material change is as yet noticed in the physical signs, the patient breathes more easily, sleep returns, and convalescence advances rapidly in the majority of instances. In unfavorable cases death may take place either from the extent of the inflammatory action, especially if the pneumonia is double, from excessive fever, from failure of the heart's action or general strength at about the period of the crisis, or again from the disease assuming from the first a low adynamic form with delirium and with scanty expectoration of greenish or pure prune appearance. Such cases are seen in persons worn out in strength, in the aged, and especially in the intemperate. Death may also take place later from abscess or gangrene of the lung; or, again, recovery may be imperfect and the disease pass into a chronic pneumonia.

The treatment of acute pneumonia, which at one time was conducted on the antiphilogistic or lowering principle, has of late years undergone a marked change; and it is now generally held that in ordinary cases very little active interference is called for, the disease tending to run its course very much as a specific fever. The employment of blood-letting once so general is now only in rare instances resorted to; but, just as in pleurisy, pain and difficulty of breathing may sometimes be relieved by the application of a few leeches to the affected side. In severe cases the cautious employment of aconite or antimony at the outset appears useful in diminishing the force of the inflammatory action. Warm applications in the form of poultices to the chest give comfort in many cases. Cough is relieved by expectorants, of which those containing carbonate of ammonia are speciall usefuly. Any tendency to excessive fever may often be held in check by quinine. The patient should be fed milk, soups, and other light forms of nourishment. In the latter period of the disease stimulants may be called for, but most reliance is to be placed on nutritious aliment. After the acute symptoms disappear counter irritation by iodine or a blister will often prove of service in promoting the absorption of the inflammatory products. After recovery is complete the health should for some time be watched with care.

When pneumonia is complicated with any other ailment or itself complicated some pre-existing malady, it must be dealt with on principles applicable to these conditions as they may affect the individual case.

Catarrhal or Lobar Pneumonia (*Bronchi* pneumonia) differs from the last in several important pathological and clinical points. Here the inflammation is more diffuse and tends to affect lobules of lung tissue here and there, rather than one more lobe as in croupous pneumonia. At first the affected patches are dense, non-crepitant, with a bluish red appearance tending to become gray or yellow. Under the microscope the air vessels and finer bronchi are crowded with cells, the result of the inflammatory process, but there is no fibrinous exudation such as is present in croupous pneumonia. In favorable cases resolution takes place by fatty degeneration, liquefaction, and absorption of the cells; but on the other hand they may undergo caseous degenerative changes, abscesses may form, or a condition of chronic interstitial pneumonia be developed, in both of which cases the condition passes into one of phthisis. Evidence of previous bronchitis is usually present in the lungs affected with catarrhal pneumonia. In the great majority of instances catarrhal pneumonia occurs as an accompaniment or sequel of bronchitis either from the inflammation passing from the finer bronchi to the pulmonary air vessels, or from its affecting portions of lung which have undergone collapse. It occurs most frequently in children, and is often connected with some pre-existing acute ailment in which the bronchi are implicated, such as measles or whooping cough. It likewise affects adults and aged people in a more chronic form as the result of bronchitis. Sometimes a condition of catarrhal pneumonia may be set up by the plugging of one or more branches of the pulmonary artery, as may occur in heart disease, pyæmia, etc.

The symptoms characterizing the onset of catarrhal pneumonia in its more acute form are the occurance during an attack of bronchitis of a sudden and marked elevation of temperature, together with a quickened pulse and increased difficulty in breathing. The cough becomes short and painful, and there is little or no expectoration. The physical signs are not distinct, being mixed up with those of the antecedent bronchitis; but should the pneumonia be extensive there may be an impaired percussion note with tubular breathing and some bronchophony.

Acute catarrhal pneumonia must be regarded as a condition of serious import. It is apt to run rapidly to a fatal termination, but on the other hand a favorable result is not unfrequent if it is recognized in time to admit of efficient treatment. In the more chronic form it tends to assume the characters of chronic phthisis. The treatment is essentially that for the more severe forms of bronchitis were in addition to expectorants together with ammoniacal, ethereal, and alcoholic stimulants, the maintenance of the strength by good nourishment and tonics is clearly indicated. The breathing may often be relieved by light, warm applications to the chest and back. Convalescence is often prolonged, and special care will always be required in view of the tendency of the disease to develop into phthisis.

Chronic Interstitial Pneumonia or Cirrhosis of the lung is a slow, inflammatory change affecting chiefly one portion of the lung texture, viz: its fibrous stroma.

The changes produced in the lung by this disease are marked chiefly by the growth of nucleated fibroid tissue around the walls of the bronchi and vessels, and in the intervesicular septa, which proceeds to such an extent as to invade and obliterate the air cells. The lung, which is at first enlarged becomes shrunken, dence in texture, and solid, any unaffected portions being emphysematous; the bronchi are dilated, the pleura thickened, and the lung substance often deeply pigmented, especially in the case of miners, who are apt to suffer from this disease. In its later stage the lung breaks down, and cavities form in its substance as in ordinary phthisis.

This condition is usually present to a greater or less degree in almost all chronic diseases of the lungs and bronchi, but it is especially apt to arise in an extensive form from pre-existing catarrhal pneumonia and not infrequently occurs in connection with occupations which necessitate the habitual inhalation of particles of dust, such as those of colliers, flax-dressers, stonemasons, millers, etc.

The symptoms are very similar to those of chronic phthisis, especially increasing difficulty of breathing, particularly on exertion, cough either dry or with expectoration, sometimes copious and feted. In the case of coal miners the sputum is black from containing carbonaceous matter.

The physical signs are deficient expansion of the affected side, the disease being mostly confined to one lung, increasing dullness on percussion, tubular breathing, and moist sounds. As the disease progresses retraction of the side becomes manifest, and the heart and liver may be displaced. Ultimately the condition both as regards physical signs and symptoms takes the characters of the later stages of phthisis with colliquative symptoms, increasing emaciation, and death. Occasionally dropsy is present from the heart becoming affected in the course of the disease. The malady is of usually long duration, many cases remaining for years in a stationary condition and even undergoing temporary improvement in mild weather, but the tendency is on the whole downward.

The treatment is conducted on similar principles to those applicable in the case of phthisis. Should the malady be connected with a particular occupation, the disease might be averted or at least greatly modified by early withdrawal from such source of irritation.

No person can when convalescent from an attack of pneumonia or la grippe say that they are free from all its ravages, as in many cases it leaves the system in an imporverished condition, and in fact the blood still contains the bacilli; and it behooves the patient to place themselves under the St. Philip's Special Remedies Co.'s care to entirely eradicate the germs of the disease, for if not entirely eradicated is liable to become chronic and simptoms of the malady will make its appearance fall and spring time, sometimes in a mild way and again in a malignant form.

The Clancy Discoveries which are administered by the St. Philip's Special Remedy Co. will strengthen the respiratory organ and lymphatic gland and intercostal muscles, and increase the red corpuscles, also neutralize the blood and restore its healthy color.

CHAPTER X.

WHAT CONSTITUTES BRIGHT'S DISEASE.

A MORBID condition of the Urine, symptomatic of Renal Disease, but not always consequent on it, and characterized by the presence of Albumen.

Albuminuria is not Bright's Disease. It is always associated with it, but may exist prior to and independently of any renal disease. If neither blood nor pus be present in the urine, but if nevertheless it be coagulable in even a considerable degree, thereby indicating the presence of albumen, it does not follow that there is any structural change in the substance of the gland. Albuminuria is frequently of neurotic origin, is a symptom of Exophthalmic Bronchocele, and sometimes consequent on cold bathing.

DIAGNOSIS.—Dr. Roberts has shown how to determine whether albuminuria be consequent on renal disease by ascertaining (1) the temporary or persistent duration of the albuminuria; (2) the quantity of albumen present and the occurrence and character of a deposit of renal derivatives; (3) the presence or absence of any disease outside the kidneys which will account for the albuminuria. Though albumen is not a constituent of healthy urine, it may exist in the urine of healthy persons, or of persons whose health is only slightly and temporarily disordered.

SYMPTOMS.—The quantity, density, and color of the urine remaining at a healthy standard, the tests by heat and nitric acid shows intermittent coagulability.

CAUSES.—Febrile and inflammatory diseases; visceral disease, neurotic irritation; dyspepsia; excessive albuminous diet, such as eggs; bathing in cold water may produce transient albumonuria; and if such bathing be frequently repeated the consequent repression of cutaneous secretion may lead to increased blood pressure in the internal organs and produce permanent mischief and structural degeneration of the kidney. It is probable that active swimmers are less likely to suffer than occasional bathers.

Nephritis is inflammation of the kidneys, producing a morbid condition of the gland and its secretions.

Bright's Disease is a morbid condition of the kidneys; the term is "generic," and includes several forms of acute and chronic diseases of the kidney, usually associated with albumen in the urine, and frequently with dropsy and with various secondary diseases resulting from deterioration of the blood.

ACUTE NEPHRITIS.

ACUTE BRIGHT'S DISEASE.

SYMPTOMS.—Anasarce of the upper as well as the lower parts of the body; the hands and feet as well as the face being puffy and swollen; febrile symptoms, a dry harsh skin, quick hard pulse, thirst, and often sickness from sympathy of the stomach with the kidneys. The skin is tense with the infitration of serous fluid through the subcutaneous areolar tissue, but it does not pit. There is frequent desire to pass water, which is scanty, highly colored or smoky looking albuminous and of high specific gravity. If the urine be examined by the microscope blood corpuscles may be seen in it, and granular casts of the minute tubes of the kidney consisting of numerous speroidal tubes of ephithelium; the kidneys being in an active state of congestion, if not of inflammation. If the urine be tested by heat and nitric acid it will deposit albumen.

This condition has been called Desquamative Nephritis, owing to the rapid separation of epitheium which goes on. The morbid anatomy of the kidney shows it to be small, hard and granular.

As may be inferred from what has been stated both a chemical and microscopical examination of the urine is necessary, and should be made frequently to determine the progress or decline of the disease. Indeed, without the aid of the microscope it is often quite impossible to detect the variety and stage of the disease.

The renal symptoms are sometimes complicated with pleurisy, pericerditis, or peritonitis.

CAUSES.—The effects of fever, especially scarlet fever, exposure to wet and cold, the action of irritating drugs, alcohol, etc. Dr. G. Johnson found by analysis of two hundred cases that intoxicating drinks cause 29 per cent. of all cases, 25 per cent. are due to exposure, and 12 per cent. arise from scarlet fever. The digestive and secretory functions being impaired the blood and nervous system become deterioated, the balance blame in the circulation is lost and the secretion of the kidney is changed.

2. CHRONIC NEPHRITES.

CHRONIC BRIGHT'S DISEASE.

SYMPTOMS.—Debility, general impairment of health, and pallor of the surface coming on insidiously, with pain in the loins, and frequent desire to pass water, particularly at night, the urinary secretion being at first increased in quantity. The patient's face becomes pallid, pasty, and œdematous, so that his features are flattened, and there is loss of appetite, acid eructations, nausea, and frequent sickness, which nothing in his diet can account for. His urine is found to be of less specific gravity than natural, as shown by the depth to which the urinometer sinks below its surface; it is also albuminous and coagulable by heat and nitric acid. There is most albumen at the beginning of the disease, because the kidneys are more congested; but it is of lowest specific gravity at the end, when the urinometer may go down to 1.004, and then the quantity of urine is very small. At first the urine may be of a very dark or smoky color, from containing blood corpuscles; but afterwards it becomes paler. The morbid anatomy of the kidney shows it to be large and white.

The disease progresses slowly, but sooner or later there is anæmia, in consequence of the tenuity of the blood from loss of its albumen, so that it is incapable of producing or maintaining the floating cells characteristic of healthy blood. Œdema of the feet and ankles is present, and, in advanced stages, there may be ascites, or general dropsy. But dropsy is not invariably a very marked symptom of the disease; it is sometimes scarcely observed, death arising from uræmia—accumulation of urea in the blood from inability of the kidneys to execrete it. The urea acts as a poison on the brain, producing delirium convulsions and coma; and of coma the patient dies. Sometimes, from the poisoned state of the blood, inflammation of a serous membrane arises, especially Pericarditis or Endocarditis, setting up valveula disease of the heart, and then the patient becomes extremely dropsical, and is carried off by asphyxia, from a complication of heart and kidney disease. At this advanced stage the kidneys are found to be nearly white, or of the color of a parsnip, anæmic, sometimes enlarged and sometimes diminished in size.

CAUSES.—Chronic Nepheitis often follows acute Nephritis; sometimes it is a result of bad living, intemperance, constant exposure to wet, struma, gout.

Workers in lead, painters, and plumbers are particularly liable to the disease. It is a constitutional disease; both kidneys are equally affected, probably from some defect in assimilation or other minute changes in nutrition.

TREATMENT.—The morbid condition in the acute and chronic form of this disordered is the same. In detail, therefore, the treatment must be strictly adapted to the particularities of individual cases. The results of the remedies and means employed must be tested at regular intervals by an examination of the urine. Patience is necessary; after carefully deciding as to the line of treatment it must be steadily persevered in, as marked improvement can only be seen after considerable time.

ACCESSORY MEANS.—In the acute disease, warm baths, or vapor baths, should be had recourse to early to promote the functions of the skin, lessen the dropsy, and to carry off from the blood deleterious matters, which may be retained in it by inaction of the kidneys. Vapor baths are preferable to warm baths because they can be used at a higher temperature. The action of the bath may be much prolonged, and the bath in consequence rendered more efficacious, in the following manner: The patient is enveloped to the neck in a sheet wrung out of warm water, and three or four dry blankets are closely folded over it. He should be afterwards quickly dried and wrapped up in blankets. If there be much amæmia warm baths should be employed with discretion. Further, to favor the free action of the skin warm clothing, flannel and woolen, garments should be added, and chills and draughts guarded against. In chronic or convalescent cases, a healthy residence is necessary, including a sandy or chalky soil, and mild, dry air, so that out-of-door exercise may be taken.

Patients with symptoms of Bright's Disease should be encouraged to take abundance of open air exercise as long as strength permits, chills and fatigue being guarded against. Bathing or cold sponging, and frictions with a sheet or bath towel, tend to arrest the disease and invigorate the health.

CHAPTER XI.

BRIGHT'S DISEASE.

BRIGHT'S DISEASE, a term in medicine applied to a class of diseases of the kidneys which have as their most prominent symptom the presence of albumen in the urine, and frequently also the co-existence of dropsy. These associated symptoms in connection with kidney disease were first described in 1827 by Dr. Richard Bright. Since that period the subject has been investigated by many able physicians, and it is now well established that the symptoms above named, instead of being as was formerly supposed the result of one form of disease of the kidneys, may be dependent on various morbid conditions of those organs. Hence the term Bright's Disease, which is retained in medical nomenclature in honor of Dr. Bright, must be understood as having a generic application.

Two varieties of Bright's Disease are described, the acute and the chronic, the former representing the inflammatory and the latter the degenerative form of kidney disease.

Acute Bright's Disease (synonyms: acute, *desquamative nephritis*, acute *albuminuria*, etc.,) commonly arises from exposure to cold, from intemperance, or as a complication of certain acute diseases, such as erysipelas, diphtheria, and especially scarlet fever, of which it is one of the most frequent and serious consequences. In this form of the disease the kidneys become congested, their blood vessels being gorged with blood, while the tubules are distended and obstructed by accumulated epithelium, as also by effused blood and the products of inflammation, all which are shed off and appear in the urine on microscopic examination as casts of the systems to which the condition gives rise are usually of a severe character.

Pain in the back, vomiting, and febrile disturbance commonly usher in the attack. Dropsy, varying in degree from slight puffiness of the face to an accumulation of fluid sufficient to distend the whole body, and to occasion serious embarrassment to respiration, is a very common accompaniment. The urine is reduced in quantity, is of dark, smoky, or bloody color, and exhibits to chemical reaction the presence of a large amount of albumen, while under the microscope, blood corpuscles and casts, as above mentioned, are found in abundance.

This state of acute inflammation may be its severity, destroy life, or short of this, may be continuous, result in the establishment of one of the chronic forms of Bright's Disease. On the other hand, an arrest of the inflammatory action frequently occurs, and this is marked by the increased amount of the urine, and the gradual disappearance of its albumen and other abnormal constituents; as also by the subsidence of the dropsy and the rapid recovery of strength.

Of chronic Bright's Disease there are several forms, named according to the structural changes undergone by the kidneys. The most frequent of these is the large white kidney, which is the chronic form of the desquamative nephritis above mentioned.

Another form of chronic Bright's disease is the waxy or amyloid kidney, due to the degenerative change which affects first the blood vessels and subsequently also the tubular structure of the organ. This condition is usually found associated with some chronic ailment of an exhausting character, such as diseases of bones and other scrofulous affections, or with a generally enfeebled state of health.

It is marked by the passage of large quantities of albuminous urine, and is frequently accompanied with general dropsy, as also with diarrhœa and consequent loss of strength. A third form of chronic Bright's disease is the contracted kidney, depending on the condition known as cirrhosis in which the kidney becomes reduced in bulk, but dense in texture, from an abnormal development of their connective tissue and relative astrophy of their true structure. This form of the disease, which is commonly though not exclusively connected with a gouty constitution is apt to escape detection in its earlier stage from the more obscure character of the symptoms, there being less albuminuria and less dropsy than in the other varieties. Its later progress, however, enables it to be readily recognized. Dimness of vision due to a morbid condition of the retina, and also hypertrophy of the heart leading to fatal apoplexy, are frequent accompaniments of this form of the disease.

A fourth variety of chronic Bright's disease is described by authors on the subject, viz: fatty degeneration of the kidneys, occasionally occurring in old age and in connection with a similar degeneration or other organs.

The kidney being among the most important excretory organs of the body, it follows that when their function is interrupted, as it is alike in acute and chronic Bright's disease serious results are apt to arise from the retention in the economy of these effete matters which it is the office of the kidneys to eliminate. The blood being thus contaminated and at the same time impoverished by the draining away of its albumen from the kidneys, is rendered unfit to carry on the processes of healthy nutrition and as a consequence various secondary diseases are liable to be induced. Inflammatory affections within the chest are of frequent occurrence, but the most dangerous symptoms of all the complications of Bright's disease are the nervous symtoms which may arise at any stage, and which are ascribed to the effects of uræmic poisoning.

In the treatment of acute Bright's Disease good results are often obtained from local depletion, from warm baths, and from the careful employment of diuretics and purgatives. Chronic Bright's Disease is much less amenable to treatment, but by efforts to maintain the strength and improve the quality of the blood by strong nourishment, and at the same time by guarding against the risks of complications, life may often be prolonged in comparative comfort, and even a certain measure of improvement be experienced.

By referring to Chapter II, which explains the construction of kidneys, beyond a reasonable doubt. If the nervous system is deranged it will oftentimes affect the kidneys and produce above disease.

Also by referring to Chapter VI, on treatment of Scrofula, you will observe that the Clancy Discoveries, administered by the St. Philip's Special Remedies Company, contains the medicinal properties to remove all symptoms of above disease and restore the nervous system to normal activity.

CHAPTER XII.

ERYTHEMA.

ERYTHEMA is due to gastric disturbance or local irritation; the disease lasts about three weeks and seems to be associated with rheumatism symptoms.

Erythema, especially if chronic, is sometimes due to stomach derangements, flushing of the face after meals is a common erythema symptom; it is not infrequently caused by over-dosing with such drugs as copaiba, quinine, chloral, salicylic acid, and bromides and iodides.

Owing to the stomach and intestinal disturbance the St. Philip's Special Remedies are very efficacious by aiding digestion, and quick and permanent results follow rapidly.

ERYTHEMA, (Er-ith-e'-mah; *Epvonua*, a blush). Rose rash; a redness of the skin that may be made to disappear temporarily by pressure. E. abigne, a form of E. hyperemicum produced by the constant irritation of artificial heat. It occurs as rings and gyrate patterns on the front of the legs, and is of a deep-red color, gradually becoming browner in tint. This pigmentation is permanent. E. annulare, a form of E. multiforme in which the lesions shrink and desquamate at the center, but continue to extend at the periphery by a raised margin. It is also called E. circinatum. These rings may wander over the entire body, intersecting each other and forming elaborate figures with crescentic edges (E. gyratum). Occasionally new rings develop concentrically around older ones. The forms and varieties of color produced give rise to the name E. iris, E. bullosum. See E. vesiculosum. E. circinatum. See E. annulare, E. congestivum, E. hyperaemicum; a mere congestion of the skin; the simplest form of erythema. Swelling is absent or insignificant in the congested areas, and the tint of redness varies from the brightest red to a rosy or purple hue. E. endemicum. See Pellagra, E. epidemic. See Acrodynia. E. exudativum, and acute or sub-acute non-contagious, inflammatory skin disease, characterized by the development of symmetrically distributed raised erythematous patches, usually discrete, varying greatly in form and size, accompanied by slight transudation of blood or by copious hemorrhage into the skin, occasionally terminating as vesicles or blebs, and specially liable to relapse. This may be attended with constitutional rheumatic symptoms. E. figuratum, is marked by efflorescence in gyrate lines. E. fugax, a variety of E. hyperaemicum; it consists in a transitory redness of a patchy character, suddenly appearing on the face and trunk of young individuals and gradually disappearing in a few minutes or hours. It is frequently associated with indigestion, worms, etc. E. furfuracea, synonym of pityriasis rosea. E. gangraenosum, a term applied to spontaneous patches of superficial gangrene or ulceration seen chiefly in hysterical women. They are undoubtedly self induced, and are asymetric, usually on the left side, and in easily accessible positions. E. gyratum. See E. annulare, E. Hyperaemicum. See E. congestivum. E. induratum, a variety of E. exudativum attacking the calf of the leg immediately below more frequently than the front of the legs. It occurs either in diffuse, ill-defined patches or in nodules, bright-red at first but gradually assuming a violet hue. The nodules may be superficial or deep, a quarter of an inch to an inch or more in diameter, and may be slowly absorbed, or necrose and slough out, leaving a very indolent ulcer. The condition is most common in strumous individuals. E. interigo, interigo; eczema interigo; a chronic form of E. hyperaemicum, resulting from pressure or the rubbing together of folds of skin. It is common in infants and fat adults. E. iris Herpes iris. See E. annulare. E. keratodes, a diffuse condition of tylosis of the palms and soles. E. leve, a common skin affection, a variety of E. hyperaemicum, likely to appear upon the tense skin of dropsical parts. It may go on to dermatitis and sloughing. E. marginatum, an infrequent variety of E. multiforme, which generally begins as a flat disc a quarter or half an inch in diameter, and very rapidly enlarges at the periphery, subsiding pari passu in the center. It joins similar adjacent lesions, and in a few days traverses the circumference of a limb, or a large area on the trunk, leaving a fawn-colored pigmentation that slowly disappears. E. multiforme, E. polymorphe; a variety of E. exudativum, common in young adults of either sex, and appearing especially in spring and autumn. The eruption first appears almost invariably on the back of the hands and feet, thence spreading to the forearms and legs. In severe cases the trunk and face, and even the mucuous membranes may be affected. The lesions consist of flat or slightly convex papules sharply defined, deep-red or purplish in color, varying in size from a pin's head up, partially disappearing on pressure. This is the commonest form (E. papulatum). If the papules coalesce to form larger lesions the condition is described as E. tuberculatum. E. nodosum, dermatitis contusiformis: a further development of E.

tuberculatum. Multiple (seldom more than a dozen) raised, rosy patches, round or oval in the direction of the limb, from one-half to three inches in diameter, suddenly develop along both tibiæ, and often along the ulnar side of the forearms. They are exquisitely tender, tense and shining. The condition chiefly occurs in children and delicate young women. See Bacillus of Demme under Bacteria, Synonymatic Table of E. papulatum. See E. multiforme, E. paratrimma, the erythema that appears over a bony prominence, etc., immediately before the formation of a bed-sore. It is a variety of E. hyperaemicum, E. pellagrosum. A synonym of Pellagra, E. pernio. See Pernio. E. polymorphe. See E. multiforme, E. purpuricum, purpura thrombotica; a variety of erythema resembling peliosis rheumatica, but characterized by its erythemamatous appearance and the absence of alteration by pressure. It is attended with no general symptoms, or with slights pains in some of the joints, or with edema of the legs. E roseola of variety of E. hyperaemicum; it consists in the development of congestive patches of a delicate rose color, scarcely raised above the surface of the skin, varying in size from a split pea to a finger nail, and either diffused over the whole surface of the body or in figured groups. It is common in young children in association with digestive troubles. Its different stages have been called Roseola infantilis, aestivalis, autumnalis, annulata, but these terms are not now generally used. E. scarlatiniforme, a variety of E. hyperaemicum; it appears as a vivid punctiform eruption, sharply defined in places, attended with high temperature, often seen after injuries or surgical operations. It is followed by furfuraceous desquamation. E. scarlatiniforme desquamativum, a more pronounced form of E. scarlitiniforme, with a greater tendency to be diffuse instead of punctiform, of longer duration, and with a great liability to recur at certain seasons. The mucuous membranes are often involved and dequamation occurs in large flakes. E. simplex, a variety of E. hyperaemicum; characterized by a congestive redness of moderate intensity. It appears as diffuse or circumscribed, variously-sized lesions, which are usually not raised above the integument. It may be idiopathic or symptomatic; and if the latter brought about by a great number of external irritants, including heat and cold, etc. E. solare, E. simplex due to the heat of the sun. E. tuberculatum. See E. multiforme, E. tuberosum. Same as E. tuberculatum. E. urticans, the early or pink stage of the urticarial wheal. It is a variety of E. hyperaemicum. E. vesiculosum, the occurence of vesication in the progress of E. multiform. If the blebs are large the condition is termed E. bullosum.

CHAPTER XIII.

ERYSIPELAS.

ERYSIPELAS, a Greek word; synonym: the Rose, St. Anthony's Fire. A disease characterized by diffuse inflammation of the skin, attended with fever. Two kinds of this disorder are recognized, namely: traumatic erysipelas, which occurs in connection with some wound or external injury, and may thus affect any part of the body where such lesion may exist; and idiopathic erysipelas, in which no connection of this kind can be traced, but which appears to arise spontaneously, and most commonly affects the face and head. They are, however, essentially the same disease, and, as regards the latter variety, it is believed by some authorities that an abrasion of the skin, generally too trifling to attract attention, exists in almost every case as the starting point of the inflammatory action.

The question as to whether erysipelas is to be regarded as an eruptive fever allied to scarlet fever, measles, etc., or a local inflammatory disease of the skin, the fever being secondary, has engaged much attention; and while the weight of opinion appears to be in favor of the latter view, the facts of the contagiousness of erysipelas, its occasional appearance in an epidemic form, and the discovery in the inflamed tissues of microscopic organisms (bacteria) point to the existence of a specific poison as giving peculiar characters to this form of cutaneous inflammation. The contagiousness of erysipelas in its traumatic form is often illustrated in the surgical wards of hospitals, where, having once broken out, it is apt to spread with great rapidity, and to produce disastrous results, as well as in lying-in hospitals where its occurrence gives rise to the spread of a form of puerperal fever of virulent character. It is not so certain that the disease in its idiopathic variety is contagious to persons who have no wound or abrasion, and this form of the complaint is in general excited by exposure to cold, a predisposing cause being some deranged or low condition of the general health.

When the erysipelas is of moderate character there is simply a redness of the integument, which feels somewhat hard and thickened, and upon which there often appears small vesications. This redness, though at first circumscribed, tends to spread and affect the neighboring sound skin until an entire limb or a large area of the body may become involved in the inflammatory process. There is usually considerable pain, with heat and tingling in the affected part. As the disease advances the portions of skin first attacked become less inflamed and exhibit a yellowish appearance, which is followed by slight desquamation of the cuticle. The inflammation in general gradually disappears. Sometimes, however, it breaks out again, and passes over the area originally affected a second time. But besides the skin the subjacent tissues may become involved in the inflammation, and give rise to the formation of pus. This is termed phlegmonous erysipelas, and is much more apt to occur in connection with the traumatic variety of the disease. Occasionally the affected parts become gangerous. Certain complications are apt to arise in erysipelas affecting the surface of the body, particularly inflammation of serious membranes, such as the pericardium, pleura and peritoneum.

Erysipelas of the face, the most common form of the idiopathic variety, usually begins with symptoms of general illness, the patient feeling languid, drowsy, and sick, while frequently there is a distinct rigor followed with fever. According to some observers the fever is symptomatic of inflammation already begun in the neighboring lymphatic vessels and glands before the appearance of the disease on the skin. Sore throat is sometimes felt, but in general the first indication of the local affection is red and painful spot at the side of the nose or on one of the cheeks or ears. Occasionally it would appear that the inflammation begins in the throat, and reaches the face through the nasal fossae. The redness gradually spreads over the whole surface of the face, and is accompanied with swelling, which in the lax tissues of the cheeks and eyelids is so great that the features soon become obliterated and the countenance wears a hideous expression. Advancing over the scalp the disease may invade the neck and pass on to the trunk, but in general the inflammation remains confined to the face and head. While the disease progresses, besides the pain, tenderness, and heat of the affected parts, the constitutional symptoms are very severe. The temperature rises often to 105°, or higher, and there is great gastric disturbance. Delirium is a frequent accompaniment. The attack in general lasts for a week or ten days, during which the inflammation subsides in the parts of the skin first attacked, while it spreads onward in other directions, and after it has passed away there is as already observed some slight desquamation of the cuticle.

Although in general the termination is favorable, serious and occasionally fatal results follow from inflammation of the membranes of the brain, and in some rare instances sudden death has occurred from suffocation arising from œdema glottidis, the inflammatory action having spread into and extensively involved the throat. One attack of this disease, so far from protecting from, appears rather to predispose to others; and this fact is appealed to by those physicians who deny that erysipelas is merely one of the eruptive fevers. Such disorders, as is well known, rarely occurring a second time in the same individual.

Erysipelas occasionally assumes from the first a violent form, under which the patient sinks rapidly, and instances are on record where such attacks have proved disastrous to several persons who had been exposed to their contagion. It is sometimes a complication in certain forms of exhausting disease, such as consumption or typhoid fever, and is then to be regarded as of serious import. A very fatal form occasionally attacks new-born infants, particularly in the first four weeks of their lives. In epidemics of puerperal fever this form of erysipelas has been specially found to prevail.

The treatment of erysipelas is best conducted on the expectant system. The disease in most instances tends to a favorable termination; and beyond attention to the condition of the stomach and bowels, which may require the use of some gentle laxative, little is necessary in the way of medicine. The employment of preparations of iron in large doses is strongly recommended by many physicians. But the chief point is the administration of abundant nourishment in a light and digestible form. Of the many local applications which may be employed hot opiate formentations, such as a decoction of poppy-heads, will be found among the most soothing. Dusting the affected parts with flour or powdered starch, and wrapping it in cotton wadding is also of use; or collodion may be painted over the inflamed surface to act as a protective.

With the object of preventing the spread of the inflammation, lines drawn with some caustic material (such as common lunar caustic) beyond the circumference of the inflamed part have been supposed to be of use, but this plan often fails. In the case of phlegmonous erysipelas complicating wounds free incisions into the part are necessary.

A number of remedies have heretofore been administered at times with fair and again with indifferent success, according to the severity of the attack. As a matter of fact our cures along this line have been miraculous and the physiological action of the Clancy Discoveries that are administered by the St. Philip's Special Remedies Company justifies us in making use of the *term* SPECIFIC for this treacherous DISEASE.

CHAPTER XIV.

GENERAL DISEASES.—(Continued.)

ACUTE RHEUMATISM.

RHEUMATIC FEVER.

DEFINITION.—A specific febrile disorder, accompanied by acute inflammation of the white fibrous tissues—ligaments, tendons, sheathes of tendons, aponeuroses, fasciæ, etc.,—surrounding the joints, of which several are affected simultaneously, or in succession. The local symptoms are very erratic; the skin of the affected part is covered with a copious sour, sticky, perspiration, containing lactic acid, and the blood has a large excess of fibrine, probably to the extent of thrice the normal quantity.

Sub-acute Rheumatism is the same affection in a modified form often following upon the acute disorder.

Symptoms.—Acute Rheumatism is usually ushered in with febrile disturbances, followed by the local attack of inflammation of the fibrous structures about one or more of the larger joints—the shoulder, elbow, knee, ankle, the fibroserous covering of the valves of the heart, the pericardial sac, etc. Exposed joints appear to be more prone to attacks than those that are covered, the larger more frequently than the smaller, and the small joints of the hands more frequently than those of the feet. Sprained or otherwise injured joins are particularly liable to suffer. The general febrile condition often precedes the local inflammation one or two days; sometimes the general and local symptoms occur simultaneously, while in others the inflammation of the joints precedes the febrile condition. The affected joints are swollen, tense, surrounded by a rose colored blush, and acutely painful; pain is a more constant symptom than swelling and swelling than redness. The pain has many degrees of intensity, is generally intermittent, abates somewhat in the day, but is aggravated at night, and in all cases is increased by pressure, so that even the touch of the medical attendant or nurse, or the weight of the bed clothes can scarcely be borne. Often the patient remained fixed, as it were, in one posture, from which he cannot or dare not move. The skin is hot, covered with a sour, offensive sweat, and so highly acid as to redden litmus paper.

The perspirations, although unattended by immediate relief, are nature's mode of elimination; for the pains are always aggravated, and the constitutional symptoms intensified, if they become suppressed. It is only when the perspiration lose their peculiar sour character that they become useless. The urine in acute rheumatism is scanty, often resembling porter in color, of high specific gravity, and deposits, on cooling, deep colored sediments of urates. The pulse is round and full, varying from 90 deg. to 120 deg.; the tongue loaded with a yellowish white mucus; the head is but slightly affected. The usual absence of headache or dilirium distinguishes acute rheumatism from the continued fevers. Intense thrist is a common feature, the appetite is fastidious, and the digestive functions are seriously impaired.

METASTASIS.—Rheumatism is usually erratic; it often suddenly quits one joint to appear in another, and then in another; afterwards traveling back, perhaps to its original seat, the development of inflammation in one joint being often accompanied by its rapid subsidence in another, this alternation occurring many times during an attack. But the most serious metastasis is from the joint structures to the pericardium or the valves of the heart. This complication may be expected in very severe attacks in young persons, in women oftener than in men, in patients who have been previously weakened, and in persons troubled with irritability or palpitation of the heart.

HEART COMPLICATIONS. —When Cardiac inflammation arises, the patient's countenance becomes dreadfully anxious, the breathing distressed, and pain is complained of in the heart's region; also there is tenderness between and under the ribs, and there may be palpitation or irregular action of the heart. The physical signs of pericarditis may be detected by the stethoscope, and a distinct friction or to and fro sound like the rubbing of paper, owing to the roughening of the serus surface by effusion or fibrin. This sound may soon be lost, lost, either from the opposite surface, becoming glued together, or separated by serus effusion. If the amount of effusion be large, both the circulation and the respiration become seriously embarrassed, the heart beats tumultuously, the sound becomes muffled, and there is increased extent of dullness in the heart's region. Endocaritis may arise with pericarditis or separately. The symptoms are similar to those of pericarditis. but the physical sign is a bruit. In consequence of the extreme danger of these complications, all cases of severe rheumatic fever should be watched daily by a medical man so that the signs and symptoms of heart complications, which often come on insidiously, may be early recognized and met.

RHEUMATISM AND GOUT.—For a tabular statement of the differences between these diseases see Acute Gout.

CAUSES.—The predisposing cause is constitutional cachexia, which produces a morbid product in the blood by some unhealthy assimilation.

These materies morbi, with which the blood is loaded, constitute that predisposing cause without which it is probable the disease would never occur. Hereditary predispostion undoubtedly exists in many persons. The suppression of an eruption or rash, as measles or the sudden stoppage of dysentery, may also act as a predisposing cause.

The exciting causes are: exposure to cold and wet, especially evaporation from wet or damp clothes, causing chill. This is no doubt an explanation why the disease is most common among the poorer classes of society, who cannot protect themselves so effectually as their wealthier brethren. The cold probably excites an attack of acute rheumatism by arresting the secretory functions of the skin by means of which in health morbid substances in the blood are often removed; now, however, the functions of the skin being deranged, unhealthy principles accumulate in the blood and rheumatism results. Mere cold, however, is not so much a cause of rheumatism as extreme atmospheric vicissitudes. Hence it is found that it does not prevail most in the coldest regions of the globe, but rather in those climates and during those seasons which are damp and changeable.

DIET.—During the fever the diet should be mainly restricted to water, milk and water, barley water, gruel, and arrow-root, at least at first; afterwards, beef tea, mutton broth, etc. In rheumatic fever, a strictly non-nitrogenous diet has been found very useful. By thus temporarily cutting off the supply of nitrogenous matter, which by imperfect oxidation causes acidity, the end sought in the allopathic treatment by alkalines and by blisters is obtained, and the natural process of cure assisted. But as this diet lowers cardiac power it should be adopted with extreme caution in very debilitated patients, and discontinued if not soon found beneficial.

HYDROPATHIC.—Treatment: In the early stage of the disease is highly beneficial—Warm baths, hot air baths, or hot compresses are useful and comforting. Wet packing, repeated as often as the fever returns, and enveloping the joints which are chiefly implicated, or even the whole body with several folds of wet linen are most useful adjuncts. Except, however, when the skin is hot and dry, and temperature high, cold application are contra-indicated, as from the migratory character of the disorder, great risk would be incurred of repelling the poison into the circulating fluid, to settle possibly upon the heart or other internal part. Dr. Wilson Fox has tried with success the following treatment, which has been found especially useful when the pains were excessive and the temperature high: The patient first received a vapor bath, and then was thoroughly douched with water, commencing at a temperature of 90 deg. gradually cooled down to 40 deg. Fahr.

BLANKETS IN RHEUMATISM.—An invaluable adjunct to the measures already suggested is that of enveloping the patient in flannel blankets. Bedding in blankets greatly reduces the risk of inflammation of the heart, diminishes its intensity and danger when it does occur, and at the same time does not prolong the convalescence.

Bandaging the affected joints lessens pain, shortens the attack and secures rest.

MUSCULAR RHEUMATISM.

DEFINITION.—Pain in the muscular structures, increased by motion. The most familiar local varieties of this affection are stiff neck, lumbago and sciatica. Muscular rheumatism is rarely accompanied by redness, swelling, or other external symptoms.

STIFF NECK—CRICK IN THE NECK.

DEFINITION.—A rheumatic affection of the muscles of the side of the neck, chiefly the sterno-cleido-mastoideus, which becomes rigid, hard and swollen. The least attempt to turn the neck is attended with acute pain. Sometimes the rheumatism extends to the articulations of the clavicle and intercostal muscles.

SCIATICA.

DEFINITION.—Rheumatic inflammation of the aponeurotic parts of the glutei muscles, accompanied by gradually increasing and intense aching soreness or darting pain, extending from the nates to the knee and sometimes to the ankle. The patient is often obliged to walk very carefully, or is unable to move. Examination will probably discover no redness nor swelling anywhere, not even swelling or thickening of the nerve at the seat of pain, which is usually where a nerve branch passes through a fascia, or out of a bony canal, or lies superficially.

ACCESSORY MEANS.—Liniments, medicated with the same remedy as administered internally or even simple olive oil, rubbed into the affected parts, are very useful. The friction should be performed in a warm room, and currents of air guarded against. A wet compress, simple or medicated, greatly assist the cure. In this and other varieties of muscular rheumatism rest and warmth are of great importance. The application of the common flat iron of the laundry, as hot as can be borne, with flannel between the skin and iron, is very valuable. In lumbago, nothing is so instantaneously beneficial as strapping the back from the level of the seat upwards in layers that overlay each other, with strips of adhesive plaster or warm plaster. A pad of flannel or of unbleached cotton wool wrapped across the loins, next the skin, is very comforting. Where persons are very liable to lumbago from slight exposure to cold or damp, wearing a skein of silk around the waist is an excellent preventive. Generous nutritive diet is desirable. Lemon juice is a grateful and remedial beverage.

Rreumatism and Muscular Weakness.—Muscular rheumatism is apt to be confounded with the painful muscular affections following prolonged or excessive exertion, or with the soreness or stiffness which occurs during convalescence from any long illness or accompany general debility. These affections are generally better after the repose of the night, but increase with fatigue; and the pain in the affected part is mitigated by relaxing or supporting it.

CHRONIC RHEUMATISM.

Definition—Chronic pain, with stiffness, swelling, and possibly distortion of various joints.

This is sometimes a sequel of the acute form of Rheumatism; at other times it is a separate constitutional affection, coming on quite independently of any previous attack. It is generally very obstinate, prone to recur, and is often worse at night. In time the affected limbs lose their power of motion, and lameness results, the knee joint being often affected; sometimes there is amaciation of the muscles; sometimes permanent contraction of a limb or bony stiffness of the joint. There is but little febrile disorder, no perspiration, and less swelling than in acute rheumatism.

TREATMENT.—In the treatment of chronic rheumatism, dyspeptic symptoms often associated with it, are primary considerations and little hope of a cure can be expected till they are remedied.

ACCESSORY MEANS.—Patients who are much afflicted with this complaint should, if possible, reside in a warm, dry climate. At any rate such patients should wear flannel or other warm clothing, and guard against atmospheric changes. The feet should be protected from cold and damp. Wet compresses, covered with dry flannel, over the affected joints, are always useful. Sometimes warm baths, especially of salt water, vapor, or hot air, are most useful.

Lastly, the diet should be easy of digestion, as attacks are often occasioned by disorders of the stomach. BEER and strong wines should be avoided. Cod liver oil should be given.

CHAPTER XV.

ACUTE GOUT.

DEFINITION.—A specific febrile disease, usually occurring in paroxysms at longer or shorter intervals, characterized by non-suppurative inflammation, with considerable redness of certain joints—chiefly of the hands and feet, and especially in the first attack of the great toe—with excess of uric acid in the blood. The disease is generally hereditary, and an attack is always associated with derangement of the digestive and other organs.

SYMPTOMS—As an acute attack of gout is often occasioned by an excessive debauch, or over-fatigue, impairing the digestion, its onset commonly commences an hour or two after midnight, when indigestion from a supper or late dinner arrives at its acme. Ordinarily a patient retires to rest in his accustomed health, but awakes early in the morning with severe pain., chiefly in the metatarso-phalangeal joint of the great toe, which, on examination, is found red, hot, swollen, and so exquisitely tender that the mere weight of the bedclothes is intolerable, and even the vibration of a heavy footfall in the room causes great discomfort. The veins proceeding from the toe become turgid with blood and surrounded with more or less oedema. On the first accession of the pain there is generally cold shivering, which gradually subsides as the pain increases, and is followed by symptomatic fever. The patient is perpetually shifting his foot from place to place, and from posture to posture, finding no relief. At length, if suitable precautions are taken, and the foot kept in a horizontal posture, the pains subside in the early part of the day; but at evening an exacerbation takes place, which persists during most of the night, and subsides again toward morning, when sleep, with gentle perspiration, takes place. Sometimes the pains remit so suddenly that the patient attributed the relief to his having at last found an easy posture. The same series of symptoms recur, in a less severe form, for some days and nights, varying considerably in different cases, and being greatly influenced by the treatment adopted; and then the attack passes off, not to return for one, two, or after a first attack, perhaps for three years. After the lapse of years, however, the intervals between the attack are liable to diminish, until the patient can scarcely ever calculate upon being free. The joints of the fingers and toes become enlarged and disorganized by deposit, within and without the synovial cavity, of a white saline matter, commonly called "chalk stones," but really urate of soda.

It is not uncommon, even in a first attack of gout, for both great toes to be implicated, generally alternately, the inflammation rapidly subsiding in one joint to appear in the other, but sometimes simultaneously. In many instances, after first attacks, other joints—the instep, the ankle, the heel, or the knee—are affected at the same time; in rarer cases some joints of the upper extremities.

SYMPTOMS PRECEDING AN ATTACK.—Flatulence, heartburn, acidity, relaxed or confined bowels, and other disorders of digestion. In some patients the function of breathing is implicated, or the liver deranged, in others the nervous system is involved, with palpitation; or there may be alternation of the urinary secretion, or crampy condition of the muscles. Such symptoms are no doubt consequent on the altered state of the blood, which always exist prior to the development of a gouty paroxysm. Should any organ or function be specially implicated it is then termed irregular gout.

DIFFERENCES BETWEEN GOUT AND RHEUMATISM

GOUT.	RHEUMATISM.
1. In the earlier attacks the small joints are affected, the metatarsal joint of the great toe being chiefly implicated.	1. The large joints are chiefly implicated, several being affected at the same time.
2. Rarely occurs before puberty, and generally not till from thirty-five to fifty years of age.	2. Generally occurs in the young, from twenty to thirty years of age, and often earlier.
3. Is more frequent in men than women, and in the latter rarely till after the cessation of the menstrual function.	3. Affects men and women equally.
4. It is often the punishment of an idle, luxurious, and intemperate life.	4. Is the lot of the poor, the hard working, the exposed, and the ill-clad.
5. Is strongly hereditary.	5. Is but slightly hereditary.
6. Is associated with chalk stones in the external ear, on the tops of the fingers, or other situation.	6. Is never associated with chalk stones.
7. A fit of Gout often affords great temporary relief.	7. An attack of Rheumatism has not one redeeming feature in it.
8. Is confined to the temperate regions of the world.	8. Rheumatism appears to prevail in all climates, and has been called an ubiquitous disease.

Among the exciting causes of gout may be mentioned indigestion, especially that form of it which favors the production of an excessive amount of acidity, and tending to the insolubility and deposition of the urate of soda in the tissues. During an attack of gout, uric acid is said to be absent from the urine, the kidneys not execreting it; hence it collects in the blood, and may be detected by the microscope in minute crystals upon threads immersed in the serum, after the addition of a little hydrochloric acid.

Season and climate have much influence in exciting a paroxysm of gout. First attacks are most common in spring, as the diseased becomes more confirmed and autumnal seizure is added; after the lapse of a long time a fit may occur at any season and at most irregular intervals.

ACCESSORY MEANS.—During an attack of gout the affected limb should be raised, so as to favor the free return of blood to the heart; the application of flannels wrung out of hot water, hot bread and water poultices, after emersion in hot water, often do good; or the acetic acid lotion, before recommended, may be used. In acute attacks the patient should be restricted to farinaceous diet— arrowroot, tapioca, sago, bread, etc.—and milk; water, or toast and water, ad libitum. As the febrile symptoms decline, a more generous diet may be gradually allowed; at the same time the patient should resume daily moderate out-of-door exercise as early as he is able.

PREVENTIVE TREATMENT.—*First.* A well-chosen diet. This should include both animal and vegetable food, be adapted in quality and quantity to the ability of the stomach to digest, and at the same time furnish sufficient nourishment out of which pure blood can be formed. Soles, whiting and codfish, mutton, tender beef, fowl and game may be eaten. Salmon, veal, pork, cheese, and highly seasoned dishes are unsuitable. The consumption of animal food should be moderate, and acidity guarded against by avoiding pastry, greasy or twice-cooked meat, raw vegetables, highly seasoned food, anything likely to lead the patient to eat more than is strictly moderate. The wines most likely to injure are port, sherry and maderia. If wine be taken at all, good claret, free from sugar and acidity is best. When gout attacks a patient early, entire abstinence from all alcoholic beverages is one of the most likely measures to check its future development; but aged persons and others whose health has been much enfeebled, may be allowed a small quantity of stimulants, such as the particular circumstances of each case seem to justify.

Second. Healthy action of the skin. This should be promoted by bathing warm clothing, crash towels, bath brushes, etc., for much excrementitious matter is got rid of in this manner. Friction over the whole surface of the body is extremely useful when exercise can not be taken. The patient should be well rubbed with a flesh brush, or with the hands twice a day.

Third. Good habits. A life of indolence should be exchanged for one activity and usefulness. Exercise, not severe or exhausting, should be taken regularly. Walking so as to secure an abundance of fresh air, must ever be considered the best exercise, but it may be conjoined with riding. Without sufficient exercise, probably every other measure will be unavailing. Early and regular hours should be adopted, and severe or prolonged mental application avoided. In some cases removal to a warm and dry climate during winter and spring may ward off a subsequent attack.

CHRONIC GOUT.

DEFINITION.—A persistent constitutional affection characterized by stiffness and swelling of various joints, with deposits of urate of soda.

SYMPTOMS.—The deposits in the joints constitute the distinguishing feature; chronic stiffness and swelling of various joints, with pain, are considered as cases of Chronic Rheumatism. The original condition of the chalk-stone deposits is that of a liquid, rendered more or less opalescent from the presence of acicular crystals; as the fluid part is absorbed the consistence becomes creamy, and at last a solid concretion is produced when the effusion is confined to the cartilages, unless very execssive, the injury to the mobility of the joint is comparatively slight, but when the ligaments are infiltrated they are made rigid, and the play of the parts is consequently interfered with. If a bursa has been infiltrated, the resulting chalk stone is free and of uniform composition, but the distortion is considerable. The vissible occurence of chalk stones is not constant, but when external deposits do occur in any patient, no possible doubt can exist as to the nature of the case, for, as the deposition of urate of soda in the tissues occurs only in gout, its presence constitues a pathognomonic sign, (Garrod).

TREATMENT OF GOUTY DEPOSITS.—The following method Dr. Broadbent had found effectual: Wrap the hands in linen or flannel dripping with water, warm or cold, and enclose them in a waterproof bag all night. This very speedily removes inflammatory stiffness, and, little by little, the concretions of urate of soda soften, frequently disappearing entirely. Dr. Broadbent has, in other cases, applied alkaline solutions, and water acidulated with nitric acid, to one hand, while water alone has been applied to the other, and has come to the conclusion that water is the agent in the process of removal. Urate of soda is soluable in a sufficient quantity of water. When once deposited around the joints it is extra vascular, and not readily acted on through the blood, but water being absorbed by the skin effects its solution and when dissolved it is carried away.

The Clancy Discoveries, which are administered by The St. Philip's Special Remedies Company, are very efficacious in the treatment of above diseases, as they improve digestion and regulate circulation, also by their therapeutic properties, will expel the excess of lactic acid, also excess of fibrin.

To this latter cause, also to cold and to micro-organism, has been described the origin of the affection.

CHAPTER XVI.

From The Medical Journal of Health, July 28, 1896.

WHY CONSUMPTION REMEDIES FAIL TO CURE.

We are constantly in receipt of letters from subscribers to the Journal who have been led into purchasing speciously advertised nostrums for the cure of tuberculosis, but which utterly failed to accomplished the promised results. So frequent, indeed, have become these letters of complaint that we consider a somewhat extended reference to the subject cannot but afford interest to many who read these pages.

Why do consumption remedies fail to cure? This question may trouble the layman, but to the scientist it is of easy solution. The physician knows how detrimental to the proper treatment of a case is a wrong diagnosis, and therein lies the weakness of the many consumption remedies offered, for they start out with a wrong diagnosis, and in attempting to cure conditions which are imaginary they naturally fail. Whilst the consumptive condition is attributed to a score or more various causes by various compounders of consumption nostrums, the fact is that but one investigator in this field has come upon the true theory and has practically demonstrated its truth. Reference is had to Wm. J. Clancy, a chemist of experience and reputation, who, pursuing investigation upon original lines, succeeded in discovering the great primary physiological fact that consumption of the lungs as well as Bright's disease and rheumatism is caused by an acid condition of the blood, the disease blood in each instance attacking the organ offering the least resistance to the poison.

The toxic effect of the acid attacking the lungs causes consumption or being deposited in the joints produces rheumatism. Where the urinary organs and kidneys are weak Bright's disease naturally follows. Acting upon the knowledge obtained by years of thorough and conscientious investigation in the field of chemistry, and in demonstration of this theory evolved by patient toil and intelligent search, Mr. Clancy originated a formula which was found to be successful, that a corporation was formed and is known as The St. Philip's Special Remedies Company, with extensive offices at 1412-1413 Masonic Temple, corner State and Randolph streets.

To say that the Clancy remedy for consumption of the lungs demonstrates the truth of his theory scarcely expresses the facts as strongly as they should be stated. With this remedy have been cured scores of cases, some of such long standing that all hope of relief had been abandoned, and the corroborative proof offered must be accepted by every intelligent and unprejudiced person. Many of the most prominent and able physicians of Chicago attest to its wonderful success, and we bespeak for it a careful and unbiased investigation upon the part of the profession throughout the city. The trouble with other so-called consumption cures has been the same in all cases—their originators started out with a false diagnosis and were consequently led into errors in the treatment of the disease; upon the other hand, a success of the Clancy treatment is easily attributable to the fact that its originator intelligently diagnosed the real cause of the disease and went to work systematically upon those lines and brought forth a specific; in other words he first found out just what it was that had to be cured and then he studied out that cure. This he was enabled to do on account of his wide experience in pharmaceutical chemistry and extensive knowledge of the pathological effects of the medicinal products in the manufacture of which he was for years engaged; thus his occupation and special technical education afforded advantages not ordinarily possessed by those exploiting the numerous consumption remedies which flood the market. After the most thorough investigation, conducted by trained and trusted editorial representatives of this paper, we do not hesitate to guarantee the effectiveness of the Clancy treatment to every reader of the American Journal of Health, as we have satisfied ourselves it offers a specific cure. The number of sufferers from pulmonary consumption can scarcely be estimated. Throughout the city of Chicago may be found its victims who are lingering on without hope, for they cannot be cured by the old methods of treatment. Humanity demands that a remedy which has received recognition from every earnest and honest investigator should be availed of. There is no doubt whatever regarding the efficacy of the Clancy treatment.

We are willing to rest the prestige gained in twenty-three years of medical journalism upon the assertion that it offers a sure cure.

It is worse than folly to ignore this one hope that is offered to the victims of this painful and terrible disease

Western Trade Journal, Chicago, Ill., Aug. 4, 1896.

ANSWERS TO CORRESPONDENTS.—A subscriber writes as follows: Will you look up the St. Philip's Special Remedies Company, which claims to cure consumption. It is located at California avenue and Congress street. I would like to know if it is an incorporated company, and if so are the members responsible men? If the cure is genuine you will benefit not only myself but doubtless thousands of others by informing us. If, upon the other hand, the firm is a fraud kindly give us warning.

In response to this request we have made such examination of this corporation and its remedies and pursued inquiries among those competent to express an opinion, that the report herewith following may be relied upon by every reader of the Western Trade Journal. The company is duly and legally incorporated, and its members are of unquestioned responsibility and standing in the business world. They are men who would never lend their names to anything of a doubtful character, and the fact that they are connected with it affords sufficient indication that St. Philip's Special Remedies Company is a corporation of sterling merit, and that its object and mission is a commendable one.

We find, too, that the remedies employed by this company have been severely tested with a result of demonstrating their marvelous curative powers in consumption, and it is a subject of general remark throughout a wide scope of the residence and business districts for many blocks, radiating from where the laboratory of this company is located, that many wonderful cures have been achieved. Merchants in the vicinity do not hesitate to say that a cure for consumption has been found, and declare a steady stream of pilgrims to this one Mecca of hope pours in of mornings and afternoons, and that careful questioning of these patients convinces them that a permanent cure is achieved by these wonderful remedies.

Moreover, through our special private Enquiry Bureau, we have placed ourselves in touch with those who have been treated under this system with a result of demonstrating to our entire satisfaction that there is no reasonable doubt of the success of the system in curing consumption. We are familiar with the standing of William J. Clancy, the founder of this system and discoverer of the cure, and know that he has been connected with the special departments of pharmacy maintained by the leading packers in the preparation of pepsin and other animal products having medicinal value. An experience of years in such lines doubtless led him into investigation, terminating in the discovery of this wonderful consumption cure. Personally, he is a man of the highest standing, and his associates are strong men and trustworthy to the highest degree. We indorse the company and its cure strongly and without hesitation. There is no question whatever regarding their trustworthiness.

CHAPTER XVII.

Inter Ocean, Chicago, Sept. 4, 1896.

ASTONISHING CURES.

CONSUMPTION AND BRIGHT'S DISEASE OF THE KIDNEYS.

IMPARTIAL INVESTIGATION.

TESTIMONY OF NUMEROUS SUFFERERS IS THE PROOF.

AFFLICTED WHOM PHYSICIANS HAVE PRONOUNCED BEYOND RECOVERY SPEEDILY CURED BY TREATMENT.

Scientists have grown old and have died in their endeavors to discover some elixer of life or general tonic which would rebuild decayed tissues, reinvigorate and rejuvenate the human family.

There have been astounding revelations in the medical world which have made life easier to sustain and lessened the ills and pains of men and women. With all these evolutions of therapeutics and materia medica there have as yet remained some diseases which the skill of the practitioner has failed to control, and thousands die annually from the wasting disease of consumption and the death grip of Bright's disease of the kidneys.

Both these diseases are classed among the incurables, and the poor sufferers are advised to change climate, put on a special diet, and offered no consolation except the awful destiny of an uncertain period of death. Dr. Koch, the great German specialist, thought he had discovered an unfailing cure for consumption, and all the varieties of mineral waters from every known country have been offered to the persons afflicted with Bright's disease.

These panaceas have failed of their purpose; while contributing in no small measure to the alleviation of the suffering, still they have not proved to be general cures. Recently The Inter Ocean has had presented to its notice a remedy for the cure of consumption and Bright's disease that to all appearances after an investigation by a representative of the paper would seem to be a genuine cure.

RESULT OF CHEMICAL RESEARCH.

The remedy is supplied by The St. Philip's Special Remedies Company, corner California avenue and Congress street, and the gentlemen interested in the organization are of good standing and not of the speculative character of men usually identified with such companies. The remedy itself is the result of an exhaustive chemical research by William J. Clancy, a chemist whose attention has been directed in the abstruse problem of correct diagnosis and such a prescription of drugs as would destroy the bacilli of consumption, and supply the wasting tissues with renewed vitality.

For some time Mr. Clancy has been satisfied that his discovery was the missing link in the chain of perfect health, and his experience after numerous experiments on cases in all stages of consumption and Bright's disease has verified his theory. About ten weeks ago some Chicago gentlemen, whose attention had been called to the wonderful efficacy of the Clancy treatment, interested themselves and formed an incorporated company under the style of The St. Philip's Special Remedies Company. A building was secured and fitted up for the examination of patients, and the administering of the remedies and the work of treating the sick and suffering was begun on an extensive scale. Attached to the institution are regularly graduated physicians for the purpose of diagnosing the disease and prescribing the remedy. How successful the treatments have been se far can be best attested by the following testimonials and interviews of persons both wholly and partly cured, who freely give their names and a statement of their cases to The Inter Ocean reporter, who called to see them to verify the claims made by the interested parties of the company. The first, a letter written by the Vicar General of the Servite

Order, and who was personally interviewed and acknowledges the genuineness of the contents here given tells its own story.

Inter Ocean, Chicago, May 13, 1897.

CAN BE CURED AT LAST.

Consumption and Bright's Disease of the Kidneys.

Thorough Investigation.

What those who Suffered have to Say.

Afflicted whom Physicians have Pronounced beyond Recovery Cured by Treatment.

It has been the aim of scientists for generations to discover a medicine that will rebuild decayed tissues and reinvigorate and rejuvenate the human family. The ancients spent some time studying the question. Some few years ago the world was startled by the announcement that the elixir of life had been found by a French scientist, Dr. Brown Sequard, but the irony of fate showed itself when, a few years later, he succumbed to the inevitable and passed beyond mortal help.

Dr. Koch, the German physician, announced that he had found a cure for pulmonary tuberculosis, that dreadful disease known as consumption. Recently, in an article published widely throughout Europe and America, Dr. Koch admitted that his discovery was not what he had expected

In spite of the evolutions of therapeutics and materia, there yet remain some diseases that the skill and learning of the practitioner has failed to cure, and as a result thousands of people die annually from consumption and Bright's disease of the kidneys. In fact these diseases are classed among the incurables, the usual prescription being change of climate, a special diet, and no encouragement, but on the contrary the patient is told to wait for the slow but sure death.

Last fall the attention of the Inter-Ocean was called to a remedy here at the home that was said to be a cure for both consumption and Bright's disease. At that time this paper investigated thoroughly the cases that had been presented to it and found that those who had been treated had improved wonderfully. Deeming this an opportune time to again look the matter up and see how the sufferers have come out of the severe winter just closed, The Inter Ocean representative called on the people quoted in its article on Sept. 4 last, and found in most cases that they had been entirely cured and that one or two of the more radical cases had been benefitted so materially as to cause wonder when taken into consideration.

The remedy spoken of is that discovered by William J. Clancy, a chemist, whose attention had been directed to the abstruse problem of correct diagnosis and such a prescription of drugs as would destroy the bacilli of consumption and supply the wasting tissues with renewed vitality. Mr. Clancy made experiment and satisfied himself that his discovery was the missing link in the chain of perfect health.

A company was organized to supply the medicine to the public. This company is known as the St. Philip's Special Remedies Company, and has an office and private rooms for patients in the Masonic Temple, corner State and Randolph streets. During the past year they occupied spacious apartments in the building at the corner of Congress street and California avenue, but better to accommodate its patrons the offices were removed down town. These offices are fitted up for the examination of patients, the administering of the remedies and the work of treating the sick and suffering.

REGULAR PHYSICIANS ATTEND.

The St. Philip's Special Remedies Company insist and strictly enforce the order that the remedy shall not be given except upon the prescription of a duly qualified physician.

The following testimonial from Dr. Carey, who resides at Twenty-first street and Ashland avenue, speaks for itself:

"*To Whom it May Concern.*—This is to certify that I have examined a large number of patients before and after taking the Clancy treatment from the St. Philip's Special Remedies Company, and I am positive that a number of patient were and are cured by the Clancy treatment.

(Signed) "D. J. CAREY, M. D."

Regular graduated physicians, attached to the institution, diagnose the disease and administer the remedy.

One is assured of careful and conscientious work on the part of the attending physicians. How successful this has been can best be attested by the following testimonials, and also by interviews had with the persons both wholly and partially cured. These persons freely and willingly give their names and statement of their cases to the reporter of the Inter Ocean who called to see them.

Western Trade Journal, Aug. 31, 1897.

A GREAT DISCOVERY

In pursuance of the well-known policy which govern the editorial columns of the Western Trade Journal, representatives of the editorial corps have recently concluded an examination of the Clancy treatment, the safest, most reliable and greatest discovery ever presented to a suffering world for the cure of consumption, Bright's disease ane rheumatism and all pathological conditions calling for a safe and satisfactory specific and find it belongs to a class of preparations which have accomplished magnificent results in the way of restoring health and giving back to suffering humanity freedom from disease.

The Clancy treatment is highly recommended by all physicians as well as laymen, and is a chemical and scientific discovery of the greatest value in curing the diseases mentioned. It possesses a wider range of therapeutical properties than any other preparation of its class now before the profession. It is especially recommended for malignant cases, and gives more satisfaction and quicker relief than any other remedy.

From undisputed evidence in the hands of the editor of the Western Trade Journal, it can be said that the Clancy treatment relieves when all else fails, producing marvelous results in a short space of time, and improvement being noticeable from the beginning of the treatment; while it is not a "cure all," our investigation leads us to believe that it is one of the few remedies for consumption, Bright's disease and rheumatism that will accomplish more than is claimed for it. This treatment will not produce any depressing after effects, but it is a prompt remedy for the disease named.

The Clancy treatment is free from ingredients which often prove injurious. It contains active principles, combined with nutritive substances, which sooth and sustain, and is especially intended never to exhaust, but strengthen the weaker, as by its use every organ of the body is aided —both individually and collectively—to perform their natural functions. The Clancy treatment is easy, certain and quick in its operation, acting directly through the blood, and by its mild but searching and cleansing qualities removes all obnoxious and poisonous elements from the system and thus searching out and removing the cause of disease and suffering. Nature furnishes the work and life become pleasant and enjoyable, as originally intended by its Divine Author.

For the foregoing reasons, we feel it a public duty to give the editorial and personal indorsement of this paper to the Clancy Treatment. To such of our readers as are suffering from these all too common afflictions we advise that St. Philip's Special Remedies Company, suites 1412-1413 Masonic Temple, Chicago, be called upon or written to for such information as this article fails to supply.

Catholic New World, Chicago, March 19, 1898.

TUBERCULOSIS AND BRIGHT'S DISEASE CAN BE CURED.

In these days of much-advertised nostrums it becomes all honestly-conducted journals with the public weal at heart, rather than publicity at any price, to probe for the truth, to lay bare the animus, to distinguish between mere mercenery motives and merit and give the latter its due. Especially does this apply when human life is at stake, and more especially so when such grave subjects as consumption and Bright's disease, erstwhile deemed incurable, are to be treated.

True to the precaution of The New World in keeping constant vigil over its columns that no doubtful or unworthy object shall find expression therein, this article was penned only after careful and conscientious investigation, and therefore carries with it the unqualified endorsement of The New World. In this connection it is only just to Mr. Clancy to aver that he was earnestly solicitous that The New World should investigate and ratify the written and oral testimony tendered by the many greatful beneficiaries of this great scientific discovery, some of which is embodied in this article. This has been done in some instances by personal interview, in all cases to the entire satisfaction of The New World.

CHAPTER XVIII.

SOME HINTS ON THE REGULATION OF

DIET WITH A DIETARY FOR INVALIDS.

THE subject of food is one of deep and constant concern both to the healthy and the sick; not merely for the gratification of the taste, or even the satisfaction of the appetite, but also for the maintenance of life. In health, diet may be left very much to the inclination or taste of the individual, both with respect to quality and quantity; for unless the appetite be perverted and depraved by rich sauces and high seasonings, it is on the whole the best guide. Still, judgment must be exercised, otherwise in respect to eating and drinking man will degenerate into a mere animal. In disease, on the other hand, the appetite fails to guide and intelligence and judgment are more required for the selection and rejection of the different articles of diet; much more so, because the regulation of both quantity and quality acquires greater importance than when a person is in health. The taste of an invalid is so perverted that he may reject what is most suitable, and desire what would frequently prove injurious; and his appetite is so precarious that it is not to be trusted to regulate the appropriate quantity. Hence the severity of the disease might be increased, and the life of the patient imperilled, if taste and appetite, guided in the selection and taking food, instead of intelligent knowledge of the proprieties of the different foods, and judicious experience in their administration.

The digestibility of food and its subsequent assimilation depend, as we know as much upon the mode of its preparation as upon the condition of the person who eats it. If this be true of the "healthy" it is more intensely true of the "sick." Not unfrequently a change in the method in which food is cooked, is the simple means whereby it may be rendered acceptable, and easily digested by the individual, who previously suffered from taking it.

Such change may make all the difference for the relief of some functional disorder of the alimentary canal.

In chronic diseases of the digestive organs, in which the appetite may be unimpaired or even inordinately increased, attention to some dietetic regulation is of great importance, for in such cases there is considerable danger lest the boundaries of prudence should be overstepped in yielding to the urgent claims of appetite in taking excessive or unsuitable food.

It is almost impossible to lay down rules for the rational and methodical use of food in health and disease, for in this, as in other matters, cases must be individualized.

Sex, age, employment, condition of life, physical form, idiosyncrasies, circumstances—all are elements in the solution of the problem "what to eat and what to avoid."

No precise rules can be laid down. General principals alone can be enunciated; known scientific facts can be promulgated; well-tried common experience can be recorded; then out of the materials thus supplied the most fitting, for each case must be selected with intelligence and judgment.

There is a neglect, and even a positive violation of instructions against which we must here enter our emphatic protest. A physician prescribes certain food just as he prescribes certain medicines. But while the medicine may be honestly given, the food is withheld or other food is substituted. The patient and the friends of the patient often deceive the physician with reference to diet, and deem the original transgression and the subsequent deception quite venial offences which it is unnecessary to confess. The consequence is that the patient's recovery is retarded, and the medical man's treatment is reproached.

The impossibility of prescribing fixed regulations for diet will also be evident from a consideration of the circumstance that some person can take what others are obliged to reject. In fact, there is truth in the saying, "What is one man's meat is another man's poison." So that no dietetic rules can be laid down to suit all cases either in health or in sickness.

RELATION OF FOOD TO NUTRIMENT.

Food has been defined as a substance which, when introduced into the body, supplies material which renews some structure or maintains some vital process. Medicine modifies some vital action, but does not supply the material which sustains such action. A supply of suitable food is therefore essential during the medical treatment of disease; for medicine alone will not, and is not designed to sustain life. Neither, on the other hand, will changes of food so modify vital action when it is disordered as to render the administration of medicine superfluous. Nevertheless, it must be allowed that diet does play an important part in promoting recovery from disease, and that some kind of food does stimulate vital action in a degree far beyond the actual amount of nutritive material they supply. Food is required by the body for two chief purposes, viz: to produce and maintain the various tissues while they are fulfilling their divers vital functions, and to generate heat, without which life would cease. That the maintenance of the tissues is of great importance is evident from the decay of life, which is invariably associated with the wasting of the tissues. That the generation of heat is essential is evident from the fact that while waste of tissues may go on for a long period before death occurs, the removal or lessoning of heat is soon followed by the termination of life. When the body is in a state of disease we have, therefore, to meet these two principal requirements, the maintenance of tissue and the maintenance of heat. Now, in accordance with these requirements, there are foods which are assimilated by particular tissues and go to maintain them, called in general terms "flesh-formers;" others sustain the vital heat and are known as heat formers; others again both nourish tissue and supply heat. Food is derived from all natural sources—from earth, water and air; from solids, liquids and gases; from substances living and organic, or inanimate and inorganic The food thus variously derived is converted by the action of vital forces into those compounds which the body can assimilate and change into a part of itself. But before it can be so assimilated in the human body the greater part of it must be organic. Chemical elements uncombined are of no service as food. They must be built up into some living organism to be of service. Hence our food generally consists of animal and vegetable products, the animal having been also previously derived from the vegetable. Indeed, all our foods are primarily derived from the vegetable kingdom; for no animal has the physiological power of combining mineral elements so as to form them into food. But the vegetable assimilates inorganic materials under the influence of light, storing up in itself various elements in different combinations essential to the formation and nutriment of vegetable and animal structures. So without taking much inorganic matter directly into the system we obtain what is necessary through its presence in the organic.

All food, whether liquid or solid, may be classified as organic and inorganic. In view of their chemical composition organic foods are generally classified as nitrogenous and non-nitrogenous. Among nitrogenous foods the flesh or muscular tissue of animals contains the elements which are required for forming flesh and generating heat. Hence life could be maintained for a considerable time on animal food alone. Bread, among vegetable foods, contains nearly all the elements required for nutrition. Nitrogenous foods must all undergo the process of digestion before they can be assimilated and form part of the body. This process is really one of comminution and liquefaction. The food is reduced to a finely divided state by the action of the teeth, the muscles of the mouth, and the saliva, when it reaches the stomach, it is further disintegrated by the action of the gastric juice with which it is brought into contact by the motion of this organ. Hence it passes out in a state of fluidity, as a very soluble and diffusible product called chyle, and easily transmitted to the blood vessels. Should any portion of the food pass from the stomach undissolved, it is subjected to a supplementary digestive process in the bowel. The intestinal fluid and the pancreatic juice act as solvents; and the bile is incorporated with the food, which is now in a condition for absorption.

The primary use of nitrogenous food is to develop and renew the various tissues; its secondary use is to facilitate the absorption of non-nitrogenous food. Wherever there is life nitrogenous food must be present to sustain it; non-nitrogenous food contributes to its support; without the former the latter would be useless; the former being present the latter is a very valuable auxiliary.

Nitrogeous food is the main tissue-former, but it also to some extent produces force.

Non-nitrogenous food produces force, but it also in some measure contributes to the formation of tissue. Non-nitrogenous food comprises fats, starch and sugar, alcohol and vegetable acids.

Fat holds the highest place as a heat-former, for by its oxidation heat is generated in the system. Starch can not be assimilated without change; when raw it passes out of the system unaltered. If it is boiled the particles are ready for conversion into sugar. This conversion would take place in the mouth under the influence of saliva if the food remained there for a sufficient length of time. But it is usually swallowed at once; and when it reaches the stomach the gastric juice arrests the action of the saliva. It then passes on in a semi-fluid state to the small intestine, where the digestion really takes place. The intestinal secretion and the pancreatic juice act energetically on the starch and convert the particles into sugar.

Sugar is so easily diffused that it requires no preliminary digestive process to prepare it for assimilation. It passes without change into the circulation. If, however, it is in excess of the requirements of the system, when it reaches the stomach it undergoes lactic acid fermentation, and thus occasions the acidity from which some dyspeptics suffer; when not in excess the sugar is carried on to the liver, where it undergoes certain changes which lead us to conclude that it contributes to the production of fat, but not to the production of force.

Alcohol is very rapidly diffused through the system. Some portion is evaporated through the lungs; some is eliminated by the liver and kidneys; and the rest remains for a long time diffused through non-excreting organs when it is transmuted into new compounds. The most recent researches appear to show that alcohol yields no nutriment, but that it acts merely as a stimulant. Alcohol does not produce warmth nor sustain it. Nor does it give or sustain strength; there is muscular excitement produced at the expense of the tissue and drawing upon its reserve of force; there is, in fact, nervous stimulus, but muscular enfeeblement. When alcohol is taken in very moderate quantity it increases the activity of the circulation, causing the heart to beat faster and fuller and the arteries and arterioles to dilate, thus producing a flushing of the face; it aids digestion, excites the nervous system, and exhilarates the intellectual and emotional faculties. But the price to be paid for all this may be too high, and the habitual use of even a moderate quantity will lead slowly but surely to degenerative changes. Taken in large quantities the immediate effect of alcohol is depressing and narcotic. It alters the condition of the blood, causing arrest of chemical changes and alteration in the composition and forms of the corpuscles. Then follows an affection of the spinal cord, involving enfeeblement of nervous stimulus and a corresponding deficiency of control over certain muscles. A tottering gait is an indication of this. The brain centers are then affected, the controlling influence of the will and judgment are lost. This is followed by complete collapse of the nervous functions, the senses becoming all benumbed, and consciousness lost.

The ultimate effect of immoderate drinking is complete degeneration, and this is not confined to the notoriously intemperate or drunkards. Women accustomed to take wine would be shocked at the imputation that they were taking too much, have proved unfortunately that they really have taken to excess. The appetite is impaired, dyspepsia and sleeplessness follow. The heart is enlarged; the liver undergoes structural changes; the kidney is deteriorated by fatty modifications. The minute vessels of the lungs are relaxed and easily congested, and consumption and bronchitis result. The eyes are injured, indeed, there is not an organ that is unaffected. The brain and spinal cord and the whole nervous system suffer, giving rise to serious derangements, such as paralysis, epilepsy or insanity. And these derangements, it should be remembered, are more or less transmitted to degenerate offspring.

COMPARATIVE VALUES OF ANIMAL FOOD.

Physiological considerations and experience teach us that a mixed diet is best adapted to the requirements of the body; and that the proportion of animal food should be one-fourth, or rather more, of the total supply.

Animal food comprises (1) the different parts of animals, (2) eggs, (3) milk and its products.

The flesh of young animals is more tender than that of old, but is not so easily digested. The flesh of middle-aged animals is more nutritive, and has a fuller flavor than that of young. The flesh of old animals, though nutritive, is often tough. The larger the animal, the coarser the meat. The flesh of the female is more finely grained and delicate than that of the male. The flesh of wild animals has less fat than that of the well-fed domestic animals, but it has more flavor. The violent exercise taken before death makes the flesh very tender of animals killed in the chase.

Good meats has the following characteristics: It is neither of a pale pink color nor of a deep purple tint.

It has a marbled appearance from the ramifications of little veins of fat among the muscles.

It should be firm and elastic to the touch, and should scarcely moisten the fingers, bad meat being wet and sodden and flabby, with the fat looking like jelly or wet parchment.

It should have little or no odor, and the odor should not be disagreeable.

It should not liquefy or become very wet on standing for a day or so.

When dried at a temperature of 212 deg. it should not lose more than 75 per cent. of its weight.

It should not shrink or waste much in cooking.

Salted meat is objectionable and is unsuitable for invalids. It is deficient in nutritive value and natural flavor. It acts prejudicially on the system, by the introduction of an excessive quantity of salt and saltpetre.

Beef and *mutton* are the principal fresh meats. The former is richer in flavor, containing more iron, is more satisfying and more strengthening, but makes greater demands on the digestive powers. In many cases of illness it may be eaten with impunity, but in enteric fever it produces injurious effects. Even in the form of beef tea it often increases the irritation, keeps up the fever, and aggravates the diarrhoea. Administered in a raw state, when finely divided and reduced to a pulp, it is very useful in some derangements. It has proved very valuable in cholera infantum and dysentery when everything ealse failed.

Mutton or *mutton broth* is much to be preferred for delicate persons.

Veal and *lamb* are more galatinous, less stimulating, less nutritious and less easily digested than beef and mutton and can not be advised for the sick.

Pork, on account of its fatness, is not so easy of digestion as other meats. Bacon and ham do not so easily disagree with the stomach, but have no place in the sick room.

Venison is lean, dark-colored and savory, and is easily digested by the dyspectic and convalescent.

Gelatine, which forms the basis of soup, contains considerable nutritive matter.

Liver of the calf, lamb or pig is rich and savory, but it is not suitable for those whose digestive powers are feeble.

Sweetbread is easily digested, and when simply cooked is not unsuitable for the convalescent.

Preserved meat is not so nourishing as the same amount of properly cooked fresh beef.

Extract of meat may often prove a temporary substitute for beef tea, but it must not supersede it in the sick room.

Birds occupy an important place among the sources of food, especially in the diet of the sick room.

Poultry, such as fowl, turkey, and guinea foul, are easily digested, are milder and lesss stimulating than meat. But they are not nourshing. They contain too little fat.

Game, pheasant, partridge, grouse, woodcock, snipe and quail is strengthening, tender and easily digested. It forms a valuable diet for the sick room.

Wild Fowl is not adapted for dyspeptics and invalids.

Pigeon may be eaten with safety by the convalescent.

Fish is very valuable food if eaten as soon as possible after capture. It does not easily satisfy hunger, but is easily digested and is highly nutritious. It is especially adapted to those upon whom there are great demands for nervous energy, and is therefore useful in some cases of nervous exhaustion.

Shell fish, with the exception of oysters, are less nutritive than other kinds of fish. In some persons they produce gastric irritation and diarrhœa, and in others nettle rash and similar eruptions.

Lobster and *crab* are not suitable for those whose digestive organs are weak, and consequently should not be introduced into the sick room.

Sprawns and *shrimps* belong to the same family and are not suitable for invalids.

Turtle soup is a rich food, and, in small quantities at a time, is often very restorative to invalids.

Oysters are nutritious and readily digested even by delicate stomachs. By invalids they should be taken without the fringe or bread, and without the hard muscle by which the fish is attached to the shell; they should also be eaten raw, and masticated before they are swallowed. To eat them with vinegar is to commit a dietetic mistake. They should only be eaten from September to May.

Fresh oysters are most grateful in chronic dyspepsia, in the case of consumptives, for the trouble of morning sickness, in chronic diarrhœe; they can be eaten with advantage by the nursing mother. Convalescents from fever will find in the oyster a delicate and nourishing food.

Oyster Stew, prepared plain or with milk, and served with dry toast or plain biscuits, is excellent.

Eggs, if the shell be included, contain everything necessary for the formation and maintenance of the body. This food does not, however, exist, as in milk, in a state of perfect solution, but in a semi-liquid form; consequently some digestion is necessary before it can be assimilated. Raw and lightly boiled eggs are readily digested. If the white or albumen be coagulated by the heat of cooking, it becomes heavy and difficult of digestion. It should be particularly avoided by dyspeptics and by persons recovering from illness. A fresh raw egg, thoroughly stirred in a half pint of milk, forms, to most persons, a palatable and nourishing article of diet.

Eggs seem to be particularly useful in lung diseases, and in cases of exhaustive cough, soothe the irritable mucus membrane.

Artificial Fibrin, so called, has been found available when no other food could be taken. It is thus prepared: The whole of an egg is poured into cold water and allowed to remain for twelve hours, during which time it undergoes a chemical change, becoming solid and insoluble, assuming an opaque, snow-white appearance. This and the liquid in which it is immersed are heated to the boiling point, and the fibrin is ready for use. It is very easy to digest and in many cases the stomach will retain it when everything else is rejected, its presence creating a craving for more food, and thus promoting instead of diminishing digestion.

No egg that is not fresh is good for food, even when put into puddings.

Milk—Pure milk contains in solution, like eggs, all the elements requisite for the growth and sustenance of the body. Indeed, it may be regarded as the typical alimentary substance, for it combines nitrogenous fatty saccharine, and mineral matters, and water in such proportions as are required by the animal economy and in such a state of mixture and liquefactions as to be easily assimilated. In fact it requires no digestion, and it is this excellence which renders milk a most important and convenient article under many circumstances. In cases of fever, pure milk as the main article of diet is far superior to anything else, especially in enteric and other fevers, inducing disturbance of the stomach and bowels. Beef tea, which is commonly used, is often irritating; but milk, on the contrary, is soothing, cooling, and at the same time nourishing and strengthening. It allows the stomach to have almost absolute rest, which in many cases is all that is required. It should, however, be observed that milk would not be suitable diet, for adults in health, as the nitrogenous matter is in considerable excess in relation to the carbonaceous. It is suited to young persons who have to grow, and who in order to grow must appropriate an excess of what is nitrogenous to form a daily addition to the body. On the other hand, it is not so suitable for full-grown persons, who have not so much to form tissue as to develop heat or other force by the combustion of carbon. The constituents of milk vary in quantity and proportion in different animals, and under different circumstances in the same animal. Woman's milk is of course the standard. The milk of the Alderney cow is characterized by its richness in butter, that of the long horns by its richness in caseine. The product of young cows is preferable to that of old ones, and as food for infants that age of secretion should be less than that of the baby; that is to say, a cow with a calf two months old may do very well to feed a child of four months. The milk first drawn from the cow contain less cream than that which is last drawn. The milk of the afternoon is richer both in caseine and butter than that of the morning.

The quantity of milk may be tested by the amount of cream it produces by its weight and by its specific gravity. A quart of new milk, cooled should weigh about 2 lbs. 2¼ oz. The specific gravity of good milk ranges from 1.026 to 1.030 at a temperature of 60 deg. The addition of water or an excess of cream lowers the specific gravity.

On stale milk there is a small blue fungus, or mold, the forms speedily and soon spread to fresh milk if the vessels have not been cleansed by thorough washing with soda.

Ffteen grains of bicarbonate of soda to a quart of milk prevents it from turning sour, and also renders it more digestible.

Milk, though nourishing, does not agree with everyone. If diluted with one-third lime-water, it will rarely cause biliousness or indigestion.

Buttermilk is what is left after the extraction of butter. It of course contains less fatty matter than skim-milk but it retains the nitrogenous, saccharine and saline matter, and is therefore very nourishing and useful as an article of diet. It is one of the most refreshing summer drinks that can be taken, and is almost always allowable in sickness, especially in fevers with gastric symptoms. It appears to produce a gentle activity of the liver and kidneys.

Curds are the caseine and fat of milk combined by coagulation.

Whey is the residuary liquid after the curd has been removed, containing a little of the caseine and fat, but all the sugar and salts of milk. It is not very valuable as nutriment, but it is very digestible, is easily absorbed, and is a refreshing drink in the sick-room. There is a prevailing opinion that whey is suborific; hence wine-whey, alum-whey, etc., when the milk has been curdled by these substances, are recommended.

Condensed Milk is milk preserved by the evaporation of a large proportion of its water and the addition of cane sugar; infants thrive well upon it.

Koumiss, which is fermented mare's or cow's milk, has been found very useful in some cases of consumption.

Butter is the fatty portion of milk obtained by churning; when pure and fresh, butter is more easily asimilated by delicate stomachs than most other fats.

Cheese is the nitrogenous portion of milk with a proportion of fatty matter obtained by coagulation into curd by means of rennet. It stands very high in the scale of nutritious food; one pound being equivalent to three and a-half pounds of lean beef. Taken with bread or other vegetable diet it is very nutritive to persons of active habits. But it is not suitable for persons of sedentary habits, or for invalids, especially at bedtime.

CHAPTER XIX.

VEGETABLE FOOD.

Vegetable products enter largly into the food of man. Farinaceous seeds form the largest portion of our vegetable food and are of great nutritive value.

Cereals hold the first place. The general composition of all is very similar, but on account of the difference that exists in the proportions of their component elements they have different nutritive values. On an average wheat contains more nitrogenous matter than other grains. Oats come nearest to wheat in this respect.

Corn is rich in fatty matter, moderately so in nitrogenous, but poor in salts.

Rice is very rich in starch, but poor in other constituents.

Wheat corresponds more nearly to the requirements of the human system under ordinary circumstances than any other grain. As it is ordinarily used, however, it is deprived of much of its nutritive value, for the portion which contains the largest amount of nitrogenous matter is removed in order to meet the demand for whiteness in the bread. Each grain, after being threshed out of the straw and winnowed from the husks, is composed of a hard, thin outer coat, or bran, a soft friable intermediate layer of cells, and a central white substance chiefly composed of starch. The outer coat is woody, indigestible, useless for nutrition, and irritating to the alimentary canal. For invalids and persons whose digestive organs are in a state of susceptibility it is too irritating. The inner coat is of most value. It is usually removed with the outer coat in dressing flour. But it is the richest part of the grain, the part which contains food for muscles, bones and brains; and the more thoroughly this is removed, the finer the flour is dressed, the whiter the bread produced, the less valuable is the bread for nutrition. Central white material of the grain is chiefly composed of starch. but it comprises also a proportion of the more nourishing elements. Many writers have pointed out the unwisdom of preferring white bread to that which contains the nitrogenous portion. Certainly to most persons the white bread is more palatable, and presents a more pleasing appearance. It would be better to sacrifice the appearance and cultivate another taste, if thereby more nutriment could be obtained.

Young and growing children are great but unconscious sufferers from the common custom. Many are weak from malnutrition, grow up with defective teeth and bones, weak tissues, inadequate muscular development, and are susceptible to diseases which they have not constitutional strength to combat and resist.

Bread made with sea water is said to increase the appetite and stimulate digestion.

Stale bread is preferable to new; it is more friable under action of the teeth and more easily penetrated by the digestive juices than new bread. It is generally the most digestible one or two days after it has been baked.

Aerated bread, made by forcing pure carbonic acid into the dough, keep better than other kinds, is free from yeast, does not induce fermentative changes in the stomach, which causes dyspepsia, flatulence and heartburn.

As bread made of white flour is pure in fats and salts, the common practice of eating butter or other fat with it is therefore more than the gratification of a taste, it is a physiological necessity.

Toasting bread greatly increases its digestibility, provided the process be properly carried out. To cut the slices so thick that while the sides are rendered crisp, the interior becomes spongy, and then to soak the whole with butter is to render toast very indigestible. The slice should be toasted brown, not burnt, so that it may be crisp and firm throughout. It then constitutes the best form in which starchy food can be given; for much of the starch is changed into glucose by the heat. The butter should be applied as the toast is eaten, so that it may not become soaked with the butter.

Toast water, when properly prepared, forms an almost indispensable article in the sick-room.

Biscuit powder, made from ship biscuits, which consist of flour and water only, and prepared with milk, can be sometimes taken by invalids who cannot bear solid food.

Cracknells are light, and easily digested.

Sponge cakes are also light and often tempting. They may be soaked in hot milk.

Macaronni and *vermicilli* are very nutritious, but not easily digested on account of the closeness of their tecture.

Oats, when ground, form a very nutritious food. When deprived of their covering oats are known as groats or grits; groats and milk furnish perfect nourishment, even for an adult.

Porridge is a hasty pudding of boiled oatmeal. Oatmeal in all its forms is somewhat laxative, and often causes irritation of the bowels, especially if not sufficiently cooked. There are some persons who cannot take it on account of the acidity and eructation which it causes.

Barley is not so much employed as it used to be in the form of bread. The best way to use barley flour is in the form of gruel. The nutritive value of barley is somewhat inferior to wheat. Malt is rarely changed in the process of manufacture, so that a peculiar active nitrogenous principle, called diastase, is developed, which has the power of converting starch into dextrine and sugar.

An *infusion of malt* is made by boiling four tablespoonfuls of ground malt in a pint of water for ten minutes. The liquid is drained off, diluted one-half with milk or given pure. It is very agreeable and nutritious, and is often beneficial in some cases of cholera infantum, when other things are rejected.

Rye is more like wheat than other cereals in its fitness for making bread; but it is not so nutritious as wheaten bread, while its color and acidity render it distasteful to some. It possesses laxative properties.

Indian Corn, or maize, is not adapted for the manufacture of bread on account of its deficiency in gluten, unless wheat or rye flour be mixed with it. The large proportion of fatty matter, nevertheless, renders it very nutritious.

Rice is said to be the food of nearly one-third of the human race. It is useful as an article of diet whether whole or ground. It should be thoroughly cooked. In India rice is never prepared alone, but always with the addition of a certain pulse which abounds in albuminates. Rice, boiled or baked with milk and eggs as pudding, forms a substantial meal.

Rice-Water is very useful as a drink in all irritable states of the alimentary tract, as in dysintery and diarrhœa.

Of the various farinaceous preparations adapted to the digestive powers of infants, dyspeptics, and invalids generally, Neave's, Ridge's, and Hard's take the lead, and each of these has its recommendations. We give the preference to Neave's, so long as it is obtained fresh and in good condition.

Passing now to the products of the kitchen gardens, classified according to the chief purposes they subserve in the animal economy, and its average value.

Starchy and Sugary Plants.—Potatoes, yams, chestnuts, beans, lentils, peas, artichokes, carrots, parsnips, beets, salsify, turnips. Each of these is a force-giver, but each may be unsuitable for food in some disordered conditions.

Stimulants.—Asparagus, onions, garlic, aromatic herbs, mustard, cress, and a few other pungent salad materials. These cause increased secretion of saliva and gastric juice, and thus promote the digestion of a larger quantity of food than could otherwise be dissolved.

Anti-Scorbutics.—Cabbages, tomatoes, and salad materials in general. These products contribute valuable saline materials to the blood; but they should be quite fresh or they will cause indigestion.

Diluents. — Cabbages, spinach, wintergreens, cauliflower, sorrel, or any leaves sufficiently palatable to eat and soft to swallow, and which are green when boiled. The chief uses of these is to render other food more thoroughly open to the action of digestive secretions. Though not apparently nutritious in themselves they make other things nutritious.

Potatoes are an agreeable and wholesome article of food, easily cultivated, easily cooked, but not always easily digested. The proportion of starchy constituents is large, and of nitrogenous elements small, so that it is desirable to eat with them some other food, such as meat, fish, bacon, buttermilk, etc., in order that a fully nutritious diet may be supplied.

Preparation for the Table.—The best method of cooking potatoes is by steaming them in the skin; by this process heat penetrates everywhere, and there is no loss of material and salts. If the potatoes are boiled the skins should not be previously removed, or a large amount of salts will pass out. The addition of common table salt to the water is advantageous, for it helps to retain the natural salts.

Roasted potatoes are more nutritious than boiled. Potatoes are spoiled by germination and by frost.

Carrots make a pleasant change in one vegetable fare, but are apt in some cases to produce flatulence.

The *Parsnip* possesses the same general character as the carrot.

The *Turnip* contains a very large proportion of water, and hence is of little nutritive value, and is more difficult of digestion than carrots or parsnips.

Radishes are somewhat like the turnip, but being usually eaten raw, are often indigestible.

We now turn to another class of vegetables. The leaves, shoots, and stems of some plants are valuable for food, chiefly on account of the salts they contain, and because they give variety to the diet. Green vegetables are always more or less relaxing, and possess a high anti-scorbutic value. In all cases they should be eaten as fresh as possible, otherwise they will ferment in the stomach and cause flatulence.

Cabbages, *Savoys*, *Sprouts*, *Cauliflower*, etc., are of the same general character; they contain but little nutrition and are not easy of digestion, and, therefore, not suitable for dyspeptics, while the large proportion of sulphur they contain causes disagreeable flatulence of corbonic acid and sulphuretted hydrogen. Cabbage, however, is a most valuable anti-scorbutic, but if fermentation has begun its virtue is destroyed.

Spinach is wholesome and somewhat laxative.

Rhubarb is eaten as a fruit rather than as a vegetable, and requires to be well sweetened to make it palatable. As it contains oxalate of lime, it should be avoided by those who are subject to calculus.

Celery is sweet and mild when well cultivated, (and is thought by some to act as a sedative, quieting the nerves). Used in soups it is delicious and wholesome.

Asparagus should be eaten as soon as possible after being cut. The greenest heads are to be preferred, as they contain the largest amount of the peculiar principles of the plant. There need be no fear that they will prove injurious to the kidneys. Slight cases of rheumatism have been cured by eating freely of this plant; and chronic cases of rheumatic gout and gravel much relieved.

Onions are very wholesome vegetables, whether eaten raw, stewed, or roasted; they are too strong, however, for invalids when they have not been cooked, and some cannot eat them raw or cooked.

Lettuce is agreeable, cooling and digestible as a salad; the juice is mildly soporific.

Cucumbers eaten raw and quite fresh at the beginning of a light meal may be indulged in by some with impunity; but they are indigestible and apt to disagree with many persons.

Squashes and *Pumpkins* contain much water but little nutriment; they are easily digested.

Mushrooms, which are generally eaten after being stewed, sometimes disagree with dyspeptics, and had best be avoided, for sometimes they cause colic, vomiting and purging. Those mushrooms grown in open pastures are by far the best. It is not always easy to distinguish mushrooms from poisonous fungi, so that some caution is desirable in gathering them and preparing them for food.

A meadow mushroom should peel easy, and it should be of a clean pink color inside, like a baby's hand, and have a frill attached to the stalk. When the gills are brown they are growing old and dry and losing their nutritive qualities.

Vegetable Broths, made of any of the ordinary market vegetables in season, by boiling and straining, are useful as substitutes for animal foods when the latter are not allowed. Out of season dried vegetables may sometimes answer the purpose. In preparation of these non-metallic surfaces only should be allowed to come in contact with the material employed.

Fruits are agreeable and refreshing, but as their proportion of water is high, and of nitrogenous matter low, they are of little nutritive value. When taken in moderation they are very wholesome. It is best eaten in the morning. When consumed in large quantities fruit is injurious particularly if it be unripe or overripe—in the former case by the action of the fruit-acids, in the latter by fermentation and decomposition. The seeds of all fruit and vegetables, if swallowed prove more or less irritating to the intestines, and in inflamed or ulcerated conditions may do irreparable mischief.

Apples, when raw, are not easily digested; when cooked, are light, digestible and wholesome. Roasted apples are somewhat laxative, and may be eaten to counteract constipation.

Pears, when ripe, are more digestible than apples, but as they decay sooner they are more likely to produce derangements of the bowels.

The *Orange* is one of the most agreeable and useful fruits for the sick-room. It is less likely to cause disorder than most other fruits.

The *Lemon* is too acid to be eaten alone. The juice is beneficial in rheumatic affections, but in the form of lemonade it makes a cooling and refreshing drink. Lemon juice is very valuable as an anti-scorbutic; so also is lime-juice.

Plums are less wholesome than most other fruits; when cooked there is less objection to them.

Cherries, also, when unripe or overripe, disorder the bowels.

Peaches, *Nectarines* and *Apricots* are luscious fruits when quite ripe, yielding a delicious pulp for the refreshment of the invalid; the skin should be rejected.

Grapes are most refreshing, wholesome and nutritious in the sick-room when ripe and not decayed; the skins and pips should be rejected.

Raisins, which are dried grapes, contain more sugar and less acid than ripe grapes; they are consequently more nutritious. If eaten too freely especially if the skins or pips be swallowed they are apt to disorder the stomach.

Gooseberries and *Currants* (red, black and white) are wholesome, cooling, useful fruits; but together with Raspberries are generally interdicted in acute diseases.

The *Cranberry*, *Barberry*, *Bilberry*, and *Elderberry* are too acid to be eaten raw; the first three are made into preserves, the last into wine.

The *Strawberry* is one of the most delicate, luscious and refreshing of summer fruits, and may as a rule be taken by invalids, except when diarrhœa is present.

The *Raspberry*, too, is agreeable and wholesome. So, also, is the Blackberry when in fine condition. The Mullberry is more acid, and very grateful to fever patients, but the juice only should be taken.

The *Melon* is a rich, delicious fruit, but not unfrequently disagrees with those whose digestive powers are weak. The Pineapple should not be eaten by invalids; the pulps should be rejected if the juice be taken.

The *Fig* is sweet and nourishing; its pulp may be eaten by invalids, but if eaten too freely will irritate and disorder the bowels; the skin is rather indigestible.

Tamarinds are cooling and laxative, and when mixed with milk to produce tamarind whey, form an agreeable drink for febrile cases.

Olives.—The so-called Spanish are the best, being soft, pulpy and oily. Olive oil is regarded the most digestible of fatty foods, even more so than fresh butter. It should, however, be thoroughly good, pale, clear and free from rancid smell to justify this estimate. Lucca oil, with its nutty odor, is the best.

Gum is the solidified juice which exude through the bark of trees. Gum arabic, which flows from the accacia in Arabia, Egypt, etc., is what is usually employed in the preparation of drinks.

Seaweeds are among the most nitrogenous of vegetable products; in fact they are richer in nitrogenous matter than oatmeal or indian corn. It is much to be regretted that they are so much neglected.

Sugar is an important alimentary product, chiefly found in the vegetable kingdom. It also exists in the animal economy and is there known as the sugar of milk. The vegetable sugar exists in two varieties—cane sugar and grape sugar. Grape sugar, or glucose, is inferior in sweetness and crystallizing power, and abound in grapes and other fruits and vegetables. It may be obtained by chemical change from cane sugar, starch, gum, corn, etc. Sugar is valuable from a dietetic point of view, not only as rendering more palatable many articles of food, but also as productive of fat and force. As it is readily dissolved and diffused it requres no preliminary digestion in order that it may be absorbed through the mucous membranes. In ordinary cases it does not, therefore, occasion any gastric derangement; but when taken in excess or by some dyspeptics it is liable to undergo acid fermentation, and occasion acidity and flatulence. Sugar of milk does not undergo this change.

Treacle and *Molasses* are the respective uncrystallized residue drained from refined and raw sugar.

Golden Syrup is treacle purified by being reboiled and filtered through animal charcoal. If largely taken these products are laxative. They are appropriately taken with all kinds of farinaceous foods, such as puddings and porridge, etc.

Honey is a concentrated sugar mixed with odorous coloring, gummy and waxy matters gathered from flowers by the bee for its own consumption, but undergoing some modification by the secretion of the insect. It is of the same dietetic value as sugar.

Manna is a solidified juice of some species of ash, containing a peculiar saccharine principle—sweet, odorless, crystallizable—white, but differing from sugar in that it does not undergo alcoholic fermentation when brought into contact with yeast. It is chiefly used as a mild and safe laxative, but it is also nutritive.

Such condiments as vinegar, salt, and pepper are of real dietetic value, as they make the food more tempting to the palate, stimulate a flagging appetite, assist digestion by promoting the flow of secretions and the movements of the alimentary canal and counteract the action of injurious ingredients of food. Excessive use of them, however, promotes indigestion and they are of less value in the sick-room, salt excepted. The constant presence of this mineral in the secretions and the necessity for it in due proportions in the blood, indicate the importance of a proper supply with the food. This is evident in the instinctive desire of animals and in our own craving for it when it is not supplied in sufficient quantity.

Vinegar is useful in helping the stomach to digest both animal and vegetable food, particularly if the fibre is somewhat hard and difficult to break up. It is, therefore, the fitting accessory to such animal food as invalids should banish from their table, but it can be made use of by those of weak digestion when they wish to vary their diet with a cool salad.

Both cayenne and black pepper by stimulating the flow of gastric juice are valuable aids to digestion when used with discretion.

CHAPTER XX.

LIQUIDS.

Water.—There is no beverage so wholesome or to the unperverted taste so agreeable as pure water, the natural drink of man, which may always be taken in moderation when thirst is present. In some form or other it is essential to life. Water is requisite in in many function of animal economy for exemple it favors digestion by promoting the solution of our food, and acts as a vehicle to convey the more dense and less fluid substances from the stomach to their destinations in the body. It gives fluidity to the blood, holding in suspension or solution the red globules, fibrin, albumen and all the various substances which enter into the different structures, for the whole body is formed from the blood. Water enters into the composition of the tissues of the body, lubricates those tissues, and forms a necessary part of our bodily structure. It equalizes the temperature of the body by evaporation, and regulates the chemical changes resulting from nutrition and delay. It is the vehicle for the removal of effete products from the body; increased water drinking causes increased flow of urine, and thereby facilitates the excretion of solid particles. In this way some of the impurities which causes gout, gravel, etc., may be eliminated.

It has been supposed that water should not be taken with meals; but this is an error. An excessive quantity might prove prejudicial. Water is the same substance from whatever source derived. When allusion is made to differences between waters it is really to various bodies mingled with the waters. Thus a water analysis really means an analysis of the foreign bodies held in suspension by the water. Water is sometimes hard and sometimes soft, according to the appearance or non-appearance of soap-bubbles when washing. Generally speaking, the difference depends upon the carbonate of lime held in solution; until this is exhausted soap-bubbles or lather can not be produced. Hardness is due to the presence of magnesia as well as lime. Carbonate of lime in small proportion in drinking water is not injurious to most persons. Indeed, there is evidence to show that is assimilated, and aids in the formation of the phosphate of lime in bones; it is therefore useful for rickety children.

Rainwater is soft and naturally contains the largest amount of solid, impurity, but unless carefully collected and kept covered is likely to become impure.

Spring Water is rain water which has percolated through the earth and acquired saline elements from the soil through which it has passed. Chalybeate and other mineral waters are thus charged and should be taken only when prescribed as therapeutic agents.

Well Water is collected spring water. If the well be deep, and there be no leakage into it from some higher layer of soil, or from some neighboring decaying animal or vegetable matters, it usually affords a safe and wholesome drink.

Some of the purest water is obtained from deep wells bored through the earth and clay to the chalk. Superficial well water, however clear, bright and tasteless, should be regarded with suspicion, for it is frequently saturated with leakage from privies, drains, or cess-pools often covered up unknown.

River Water is partly rain-water and partly spring-water, subject to impurity from the soil, and from decaying vegetable and animal matters, and, therefore, useful only to a limited extent. The flow of the stream and the absorbing influence of vegetation tend to purify the water by oxidation.

Distilled Water is pure, but insipid from its lack of air; its softness makes it easily susceptible to the action of lead; but it is excellent for making tea or other infusions.

Water may be impure from an excess of saline ingredients, from the presence of organic impurities, or from contamination with lead. The chief danger to health is from organic impurity. Cholera and enteric fever have been traced to drinking impure water. Lead contaminates pure water, but if there be a moderate quantity of earthy salts in the water they form an insoluble incrustation in the pipes, which is protective.

It is most important that the receptacles for water-tanks and cisterns should be carefully examined and thoroughly cleansed at regular seasons, especially after a time of drought and before the approach of winter. The deleterious consequences that ensue from neglect of this duty are often alarming, although the source of evil be unsuspected. Boiling water removes some of the salts from hard water and destroys the activity of any organic impurities. Filtration through charcoal also purifies the water by removing organic matters; but a filter, to be effective, must be frequently cleansed.

Water may be administered to patients at any temperature that may be desired, but if very cold the quantity should be very small, for in some diseases it is undesirable to lower the temperature of the internal organs. If the stomach is in such an irritable state that no liquid can be tolerated the thirst may be partially allayed by sucking small pieces of ice.

Ice is a valuable therapeutic agent, and is now extensively used both internally and externally, chiefly to check hemorrhage, to moderate inflammation and to soothe uneasy sensations in febrile and other disorders. In inflammation of the brain or its membranes, and in the severe headache of the early stages of acute fevers, it is most useful applied in small pieces, enclosed in a bladder or India rubber bag, in the form of a cap fitted to the head.

To relieve the severe pain and vomiting in cases of ulcer or cancer of the stomach, a bag containing small fragments of ice should be laid on the epigastrium. In inflammation of the tonsils, the sore throat of scarletina and other eruptive fevers, and in diphtheria, the use of ice relieves pain and arrests inflammation.

In hemorrhage ice is extremely valuable. In bleeding from the mouth, throat or nostrils ice applied directly to the bleeding vessels or to the surface, forms an efficient styptic. When hemorrhage comes from the stomach or lungs ice should be repeatedly swallowed in small pieces, for so taken it will help to contract the leaking blood-vessels.

The drinking of iced water after violent exercise is too lowering to the system, and should be avoided.

Ice is contra-indicated in conditions such as the following: Old age, especially in feeble patients; appoplexy and coma in persons with a feeble pulse; advanced stages of disease; extreme feebleness. In such cases the great sedative power of the ice might overwhelm the patient and stop the action of the enfeebled heart.

Tea is a very favorite beverage, but it affords no direct nutriment; the sugar and cream taken with it yields the nutritious elements. But though yielding no absolute aliment, tea, when taken in moderation, exhilerates, restores nervous energy, conserves force, retards the waste of tissues, enabling the food to go further in its nutritive action, and facilitates the transformation of other and particularly of fatty and farinaceous matters; the body is revived, the mind is stimulated, wakefulness is promoted and hunger is better borne. When consumed in large quantities tea act prejudicially on the nervous system.

Green tea, when genuine, is stronger than black, possesses more active properties, and is, therefore, to be used with more caution. Both kinds, when adulterated, are more or less injurious.

Tea, then, is hurtful. 1. To those of spare habits and the underfed. 2. To the young who are provided with the full amount of vital activity. 3. To those who perspire freely. 4. Early in the day, for it is then apt to increase tissue waste. 5. To nervous, hysterical subjects, or to those whose heart action is very weak.

On the other hand it is beneficial. 1. For the overfed and sedentary, for they require increased vital action. 2. For the old, whose vital activity is deficient. 3. For those who have a non-perspiring skin. 4. During the after part of the day, when the system is full of partly digested food, for thence the process of digestion requires to be quickened. 5. During excessive heat, in order to relax the skin and releave internal congestion. 6. For those whose nervous systems are firmly braced up.

When tea causes loss of appetite, palpitation of the heart, mental excitement, or sleeplessness, obviously its use should be relinquished. Tea should never be given to children.

Coffee contains the same principles of tea, and hence has an analogous influence on the system. It is, however, more heating and stimulating, heavier and more oppressive to the digestive organs, and decidedly increases the force and frequency of the pulse. Its effect upon the mental faculties, quickening the energies and causing wakefulness, is not so marked as in the use of tea. It, however, relieves hunger and fatigue, and thus unables soldiers on heavy marches to undergo ardous exertion. It appears to have a staying power, lessening the amount of waste and thus economizing other food. It is laxative to some and constipating to others, and is serviceable in warming the body in cold weather. It is also cooling in warm weather by stimulating the action of the skin. If taken in excess produces feverishness, palpitation, anxiety, deranged vision, headache, wakefulness and nervous excitement. When given strong it counteracts the effects of alcohol and of opium.

Chicory yields a drink closely allied in flavor and color to coffee. It contains no alkaloid and has no nutritive value.

Cocoa is distinguished from tea and coffee by the large amount of nutriment it contains; indeed it may be regarded as a food rather than as a refreshing beverage.

The essential principles—theo-bromide—also contains more nitrogen than theine and coffeine. The fat known as cocoa butter has this excellence, that it does not become ransid after exposure to air. But the large proportion in which this exists renders cocoa heavy and oppressive to a weak stomach, and thus unsuitable to the dyspeptic or bilious. Its very high nutritive power, however, strongly recommends it for general use. During nursing it is most useful, tending, probably more than any other beverage, to maintain an excellent supply of mother's milk.

CHAPTER XXI.

Testimonies on Tuberculosis.

A Strong Letter.

Chicago, Ill., July 11, 1896.

Monastary of Our Lady of Sorrows, No. 1432 Jackson Boulevard; St. Philip's Special Remedies Co., California avenue and Congress street, City —
Gentlemen:

It gives me pleasure to certify the following facts as my testimony to the marvelous efficacy of the Clancy remedy for the cure of consumption of the lungs.

Brother Angelo (now Father Pritzl) of this order (Servite) was declared a consumptive by Dr. Kelly, of Milwaukee, and

Dr. Hoyt, of Menomenee Falls, Wis., about two years ago, and was under treatment by them up to April last, when they announced that he was incurable. In that month I caused Brother Angelo to come to this monastery and had him examined by Dr. D. H. Cunningham of this city, who, after a thorough examination, stated that the Brother had consolidation of the right lung, could not be cured, and was a "goner." Immediately thereafter I put Brother Angelo under treatment of the Clancy remedy, and I am delighted to be able to testify that in three weeks he was entirely cured of the dread disease. That I might be assured beyond doubt that a cure had been effected, I caused the Brother to be examined by the following named physicians of this city: Dr. J. E. Reynolds, Dr. Warren and Dr. Murphy, the eminent physician and surgeon, each of whom pronounced Brother Angelo free from consumption and without a trace of consolidation. Subsequently the Brother presented himself to the above-named Dr. Kelly, who is a distinguished physician in pulmonary diseases, and was, after a thorough examination, declared cured. The Brother has since been ordained, and is now a priest of this order (Servite), entirely sound and enjoying good health.

[Signed]   Rev. B. Baldi.
Prior of the Monastery of Our Lady of Sorrows and Vicar General of the Servite Order in the United States.

Father Pritzl was seen yesterday and corroborated the statements made by Prior Baldi. He is now enjoying good health, in spite of the hard work he has recently gone through and necessary fasting during the Lenten term. On last Saturday, May 8, he was examined by Dr. C. Herman Graves, who pronounced him perfectly well.

He was again interviewed on Oct. 8, 1898, and is still enjoying good health.

Chicago, Ill., April 13, 1897.
W. J. Clancy, Esq.—*Dear Sir:*

I am pleased to state that since you have accomplished my cure in June, 1896, I have enjoyed good health, notwithstanding the inclemency of the winter weather. I have suffered no relapse of my former trouble. My lungs are better; I feel in excellent condition; I have been able to perform all the duties of my ministry since and my strength steadily increases.

Hence, for the benefit of humanity, I do not hesitate to recommend your remedy to all those who were afflicted as I was.

Thanking you for the great benefit you bestowed upon me by means of your medicine, I am yours respectfully,

REV. FR. ANGELO PRITZL, O. S. M.

Delta, Colo., Dec. 23, 1898.

W. J. CLANCY, *President:*

I safely reached my destination. I am pastor and I use a little church of my predecessor, Fr. Feriari. The people appreciate our services very much. In regard to my health, will say *I am well.*

Yours, very thankfully,

FR. A. PRITZL, O. S. M.

Postoffice box 458.

Rome, Dec. 6. 1896.

TO MR. W. J. CLANCY—*Dear Sir:*

The Rev. Fr. Baldi, of the Servite Fathers, has spoken to me of the results obtained by means of your remedy and I have wished to first experiment upon myself.

For two months I had been suffering from a terrible intestinal disease of nervous origin, at least such was the opinion of my fellow-doctors. In the course of fifteen days my sufferings were so diminished as to allow me to apply myself to my profession. Then I stopped taking the remedy; but beginning to break down, I had to commence it again.

I have found that: 1. The remedy has the power to relieve intense suffering. 2. The remedy is most efficacious in stopping the diarrhœa. 3. It acts like a tonic upon the mucus of the stomach, and facilitating the digestion, creates an appetite.

Unfortunately the lack of medicine has not allowed me to watch the effect it might have upon pulmonary diseases. At present we are treating a poor woman, to whom, as well as myself, Fr. Baldi gives the medicine with his own hands.

At my home I receive a great number of invalids, many of whom could be treated with your remedy, but unfortunately we have hardly any left.

It is but just that you should gain something, but it is also equally just that the diseased poor should be cured, or at least should be made to suffer less. It is necessary, also to send your treatment throughout the world.

To do this without injuring you the medicine could be given to persons who are known and who are honest; who would promise not to have it analyzed.

Fr. Baldi could act as your depository here, and he could administer the medicine without consigning it to anyone.

As far as the profits are concerned, things could be managed as they are in Chicago, e. g., have the patients pay as they are being treated, and then divide the earnings, or without any other obligations have us pay for the medicine which you would send to Europe. In the latter case, however, it would be necessary to send a quantity of it to try on the poor, who would then serve as advertisements.

At present it is very urgent that we should have some more of it as soon as possible, in order that the little we have to be done can be continued.

I am very sorry not to know you. Father Philip will speak to you about me. I hope that you will not deny a doctor of good will a remedy that is beneficial in curing diseases.

Believe me your obedient servant,
DR. PIETRO VINLI,
20 Via Crocifin, Rome.

Chicago, Ill., April 24, 1897.

To whom it may concern:

This is to certify that on Sept. 3d, 1896, I examined Mr. George Constanter and found the upper lobe of the right lung affected, also the lower portion of the left. I also found tubercle bacilli numerous in the sputa. He had a light fever with a rapid and weak pulse, his cough was very worrying.

I have today, April 18, 1897, again examined him and can find no trace of the former trouble; no abnormal sounds in any part of the lungs; both lungs act together; he has gained much in weight and color, and so far as I can discover is well.

Very truly,

C. HERMAN GRAVES, M. D.
Residence 289 W. 12th St.

Chicago, Ill., June 27, 1898.

To whom it may concern:

I consider it not only a pleasure but my duty to write and tell you what Wm. Clancy, President St. Philip's Special Remedies Co., has done for me.

It was said by a physician that I was attacked with bronchial tube trouble and hemorrhage of the lungs; I kept on getting worse. I changed physicians, and was examined and told to change climate, as I could not be cured in this climate. I became so weak I could not walk a block without resting.

I was advised by a friend to go and see what W. Clancy, President of St. Philip's Special Remedies Co. could do for me, and so I did. He examined me and said that it was consumption I had. I started at once to take his medicine, and found I was getting better, and in ten days I could do light work. I weighed myself every day and in two weeks I had gained thirteen pounds (13 lbs.), and today I am a well man, and can't express the gratitude and joy that I feel.

Yours respectfully.

S. C. JOHNSTON,

955 W. 50th St., Chicago, Ill.

Kenosha, Wis. March 12, 1897.

Dear Sir:

I received your letter and was glad to hear from you. How are all down there? You asked me how I was and how is my health. Well, Mr. Clancy, in regard to that, I never felt better in my life. My weight is now 182 pounds, and I look good. Well, Mr. Clancy, I will be in Chicago next week and will go and see you; you can depend on that. I am traveling for the Red Star Compressed Yeast Co. now, and working every day. Well, I will close, as I have to go out and see a man down town.

I remain, yours respectfully.

FRANK E. FAY.

Subsequent letter received, Jan. 11, 1898, on file, which states his exceptional good health, at work every day, no symptoms of the dread disease.

Sept. 26, 1896.

St. Philip's Special Remedies Co., 281 California avenue, City.—GENTLEMEN:

We have today examined the sample of sputum furnished by Mr. F. E. Fay, and failed to find any trace of the tubercle bacilli.

CHARLES B. PROUTY, M. D.
D. J. CAREY, M. D.

Chicago, Ill., April 8, 1897.

MR. CLANCY—*St. Philip's Institution:*

In answer to your letter of inquiry as to my health during the winter, I am very grateful to say that my health has been very good, considering the shape I was in a year ago. I was wasted away to a shadow, as you know, but now I am as heavy as I ever was, weighing 170 pounds. Thanks to your wonderful remedies.

Yours respectfully,

W. J. SPELMAN.

7 Willis Ct., Chicago.

Engineer of West Chicago Street Railway Co., 79 W. Washington St.

April 14, 1898.

To whom it may concern:

I hereby certify that I have this day examined William Spelman, and find his lungs apparently in a normal condition.

P. J. ROWAN, M. D.
372 W. Adams St.

To whom it may concern:

In March, 1896, I was taken very sick, and after having my lungs examined by Dr. N. S. Davis, he informed me I had tuberculosis and that he could not cure me. The following June I heard of the St. Philip's Special Remedies Company and decided to take their treatment. At that time I only weighed eighty-two pounds and by the latter part of November I had gained thirty pounds.

I suffered for five months with chills, fever and night sweats and was so exhausted I could hardly walk across the floor. My friends all thought I had only a short time to live, for I could not bear anything on my stomach and I was reduced almost to a skeleton. As soon as the night-sweats stopped and the chills and fever were broken I got better, and have continued to improve steadily since, and can highly recommend the treatment to any one suffering from consumption, for if it were not for the St. Philip's Special Remedies I would be in my grave today.

AMELIA WALL,
104 N. Campbell Ave.

Aug. 20, 1898.

Rush Medical College.—J. D. Carey, M. D. City:

DEAR DOCTOR: I have examined the specimen of sputa of Miss Amelia Wall, which you brought to me, and in reply will say that I am unable to demonstrate the presence of the tubercle bacillus in this specimen. Yours very truly,

J. W. ELLIS.
Rush Laboratory.

Chicago, Ill., Oct. 1, 1898.

To whom it may concern:

It gives me pleasure to certify to the following facts relative to the marvelous efficacy of the Clancy remedies for the cure of consumption of the lungs:

In November, 1896, I was taken with hemorrhages from the lungs. Dr. James B. Herrick, (R.) Adj'ct. Prof. Med'e Rush Med. Coll., was called in and, after an examination, said I had tuberculosis of the lungs. His examination showed that the three lobes of the right lung were affected, and he said if he could stop the flow of blood and get me out of bed I must go to a more congenial climate, as medical science had as yet discovered no remedy for consumption, and my only chance was to go away. At the end of the week the hemorrhages had not stopped, although of necessity reduced in quantity.

We had heard of the Clancy remedy and concluded to give it a trial. Mr. Clancy himself came to the house; he gave me a dose of medicine in the morning, and another about 7 in the evening, and by 9 that evening the blood had entirely disappeared and *has never returned.* When I commenced the Clancy treatment I weighed not more than 90 pounds. In March, 1897, something over three months after commencing treatment, I weighed 122 pounds, a gain of about 32 pounds. In May, 1897, I had my lungs examined, and was told there was nothing the matter with them, that they were *sound.*

Very respectfully,

Mrs. Geo. F. Wood.
304 S. Sacramento Av., Chicago.

Chicago, Ill, Aug.. 4, 1898.

Mr. W. J. Clancy—*Dear Sir:* In reply to your request for a statement of the facts in my case, will say that during the week from July 27th to Aug. 3d, 1896, I was examined by six physicians (among them being Dr. Vaughan of the Michigan State University, and Dr. Arnulphy of Chicago) and all agreed that I had tuberculosis of the lungs; that I was in the last stage of the disease, and probably could only live three or four months; my temperature was 102 deg.; had no appetite and was very weak and amaciated.

I began taking your medicine, and after four and one-half months' treatment I was pronounced cured, my lungs being healed and four different physicians admitted that there was not a germ left in my system.

I sincerely recommend the Clancy treatment to any who may be suffering as I was. Very respectfully,

MRS. J. D. ALEXANDER,
3220 Vernon Ave.; Chicago, Ill.

———

MR. CLANCY—*Dear Sir:* I most heartily indorse your valuable discovery. My nephew, a child of six years of age, has taken it for tuberculosis of the spine and I feel that it has been instrumental in restoring him to health.

I cheerfully recommend the use of it to any person so afflicted.

M. F. McGUIRE,
496 Austin Ave., Chicago.

Chicago, Ill., Aug. 24, 1898.
St. Philip's Special Remedies Co.—To whom it may concern:

Two years ago I was afflicted with tuberculosis of the lungs, being in a very bad condition. I was given up by two different physicians, and after I could not retain any more medicine on my stomach was advised to go to a warmer climate. I happened to hear of Clancy Remedies from a friend of mine and concluded to try them, not having any faith in them at the time being. I had fearful chills every day for nine weeks and was so weak that I was unable to walk across a room without support. My parents and friends all thought it was only a question of a short time before I would die. To everybody's surprise I began to improve as soon as the chills were broken and today I am a well woman. I have no cough whatever, and have gained thirty pounds since taking the treatment.

After taking the treatment for one year I have been examined by Dr. Prouty and he said both of my lungs were in a good condition. I can do a great amount of work without feeling tired. I look just as robust as I ever did, and looking at me to-day nobody would believe I had the dread disease. My friends think it is a miracle that I have been cured. I feel that only for the Clancy Remedies I would be in my grave today. They only need to be tried to prove their great value.

With sincere gratitude I remain,

Respectfully,

ANNA DRABB,
675 S. Jefferson St., Chicago.

Chicago, Aug. 10, 1897.

St. Philip's Special Remedies Co., City.—
Gents:

Yours of the 6th inst. at hand and contents noted.

In reply will say, *not going over the time* when my trouble commenced, in 1891, with la grippe up to the time when I began to take the Clancy Remedies, about January 1st, 1897, but will start there. Dr. Carey made the examination and found deposits in upper half of right lung. After three weeks treatment I was examined again and found some improvement. Now, after seven months, having been examined by an eminent physician on South Side, who pronounced my lungs all right, I consider myself cured, as my feelings will attest.

Yours respectfully,

W. W. HOOBS.

Chicago, Ill., Aug. 29, 1898.

St. Philip's Special Remedies Co.—W. J. CLANCY, *President:*

It gives me pleasure to testify to the merits of the Clancy remedy, as my experience in taking it has proved everything claimed by its discoverer. I had, or at least the doctors who examined me claimed, lung trouble. I was advised to change climate, and had partially made arrangements to do so when my friends induced me to try the Clancy treatment. I was, as many others no doubt are, somewhat skeptical, and for the first few days had but little faith, but after a week or ten days saw the change and became impressed that it was the right thing, and the proper course for me to pursue, I continued the treatment with astonishishing results, gaining about 35 pounds in eight months, and in that time the cough and all other effects of the trouble were entirely eliminated. To all who are affected in a like manner I commend this remedy.

Respectfully,

A. T. WIX,

Manager Toll Lines Chicago Tel. Co.

Chicago, Ill., Aug. 7, 1897.

St. Philip's Special Remedies Co., Chicago, Ill.—GENTLEMEN:

For the benefit of that large class of humanity who are suffering from that dread disease, consumption, and laboring under the common impression that it cannot be cured and that there is no hope for them, I wish to add to my testimony to the already large list of those who have been cured by the Clancy remedy. I had been a sufferer for more than a year, and had been under the care of good physicians, but grew continually worse; finally I sent a specimen of my sputa to the University of Michigan and had a microscopical examination made to ascertain fully whether my trouble was really tuberculosis of the lungs, and was informed that it was. I had heard through a friend of the discovery of Wm. J. Clancy, and went immediately to Chicago and placed myself under his treatment, and today feel like a new man. I shall most certainly recommend it to all my friends, and will cheerfully answer any inquiries from anyone if addressed to me at Percy, Ill.

    Respectfully,
      J. R. WEEDON.

Camas, Newcastle, Limerick County, Ireland, June 11, 1898.

To Mr. W. J. Clancy, Chicago.—*Dear Sir:*

I take great pleasure in writing to you and let you know how Iv'e been getting on since I left Chicago. I got to new York and got my boat without any trouble. We sailed Saturday, April 30th, and for three days we had very fine weather; in fact we thought it was too good to last and neither did it, for the evening of the third day it got stormy and then our troubles began. Up to then no one was seasick, but next morning there was scarcely a soul on deck, so I was told, for contrary to your prediction I was very unwell myself, though I took your medicine faithfully.

Well, for the best part of three days I was in a miserable condition and couldn't eat a thing. We were seven days to an hour in the ship. We got to Queenstown Saturday about noon. The last day and a half we were in the ship a terrible fog settled on us, and try as I would I couldn't keep warm. The result was I brought an ugly cold out of the water. My trunk got mislaid and I had no medicine for five days, which gave the cold a chance to stick to me, but when I got your medicine I wasn't long getting over it. I took it steady until entirely well. I am in fine shape now. I believe myself you wouldn't know me, Mr. Clancy. I find the air here fine and bracing. I haven't weighed myself yet, but I know I gained greatly since I came here. I give your treatment full credit for having cured me.

    Respectfully,

      MICHAEL ENRIGHT.

Elgin, Ill., Jan. 27, 1898.

W. J. CLANCY, ESQ.—*Dear Sir:*

I intended writing before and tell you I escaped that dread disease, la grippe, and hope I can for the remainder of the winter. Am feeling splendid, my cough has nearly gone; do not cough hardly any unless I take a little cold; am beginning to think I am about cured; wish it was so I could get to Chicago and be examined, but am afraid to even venture as far as Elgin. If my lungs are cured would there be any need of my taking any more medicine?

    Yours truly,

      MRS. J. F. COOK.

Elgin, Ill., March 6, 1898.

Mr. Clancy—*Dear Sir:*

As it is some time since I have written to you, will now write and tell you how well I am feeling; have gained twenty pounds since you saw me. Isn't that a pretty good proof I am better? Have been doing my own work for the past three months, and you don't know how good it seems and how thankful I am. How I wish that all who are suffering as I was might hear of your medicine and find relief. Hoping to see you soon, am

Yours truly,

Mrs. J. F. Cook.

Elgin, Ill., June 26, 1898.

Mr. Clancy—*Dear Sir:*

As it is some time since I have written to you, presume you are wondering how I am. Have finished my medicine, and my cough is gone, so think I am cured, but suppose I ought to have my lungs examined, had I not? Perhaps I had better have a doctor here examine them, as I will be unable to go to Chicago for a while. Am gaining in flesh, and my friends say they never saw me look so well. All due to your medicine.

I am very grateful to you.

>   Yours very truly,
>
>   Mrs. J. F. Cook.

Chester, Ill., Aug. 30, 1898.

This is to certify that I was afflicted with lung trouble which eminent physicians pronounced consumption. In the fall of 1896 I was treated in Chicago with Clancy's Discoveries and can say to any one suffering with lung trouble that no medicine seemed to help me but this. Today I am in very good health and think it will result in a permanent cure, and would recommend the remedy to all who are afflicted with lung trouble.

>   Yours respectfully,
>
>   Mrs. A. A. Short.

Marietta, Ohio, Feb. 14, 1898.

Mr. Clancy—*Dear Sir:*

Well, Mr. Clancy, your medicine is certainly a wonder for the cure of lung trouble. I am doing splendid. My lungs are clearing up and feel nearly well. I began to improve in a few days after taking your medicine and have continued to improve right along. I am very thankful to have found a remedy that helped me so quickly.

I have a friend who saw me before I went to see you and last week he was in to see me again. He noticed the change in my condition at once and said, "Where in the world did you find a medicine that helped you improve so fast?" When I told him he said, "Write out a statement of what it has done for you. I have a friend in the American Tin Plate Mills that the doctors say must die. I want to send this statement to his brother and have them go to you and see what you can can do for him. This man has only been sick about six months. He went to California and the doctors there told him to go home as there was no help." Our object in writing his brother was to get him to meet his sick brother in Chicago.

My friend has also written to Henry Sawfield, of Toledo, advising him to go to you and get treatment.

Yours truly,
W. E. GOODRICH.

Chicago, Ill., March 13, 1897.

MR. CLANCY—*Dear Sir:*

Words cannot express my gratitude for your valuable medicine. I have taken it since last August, and I am completely restored to health and cannot omit to recommend this good medicine to all.

May God bless you.

Respectfully yours,
SISTER M. JOHN.

St. Mary's, Vigo County, Ind.,
March 13, 1897.

MR. W. J. CLANCY—*Respected Sir:*

Your letter of kind inquiry concerning my health was received yesterday, and I wish to apologize for my failure in replying by return mail, but circumstances prevented my doing so. With pleasure I assure you of the great improvement in my physical condition during the past winter. My cough has, I may say, disappeared, and I no longer experience any pain in my lungs. Thanking you for the great good your medicine has done me, and praying that many others will be benefitted by it.

I am, very respectfully yours,

SISTER ALOYSIA.

Chicago, Ill., March 12, 1897.
St. Philip's Special Remedies Co.—GENTLEMEN:

Yours of this date at hand wishing to know how my health has been this winter. I must say, physically I am not very strong, but my general health has been exceptionally good. I have not felt any pains in chest or lungs. The cough has not returned, with the exception of a few days, caused by wet feet during the heavy snow.

Yours respectfully,

JOHN J. KELLY.

Hilbert, Wis., Aug. 29, 1898.

Dr. W. J. Clancy, Chicago—*Dear Sir:*

Now that there is nearly one year elapsed since I began to take your medicine I feel as though I should give you an accurate account of the symtoms and condition of my health. In comparison to a year ago I must candidly confess that my condition has greatly improved, as so my voice. I can gladly state that it is quite distinct and clear again save on misty, damp and rainy weather. As to the cough I can state that I am not troubled any more save in the morning when it is cold or chilly. My expectoration is very little and only when I must cough. My lungs seems to be improved although yet I feel occasionally the depression in right lung.

I do not feel the indescribable sensation or pain in the neighborhood of the heart save once in a great while, however does not yet beat normal.

As to weight I must say I gained nothing or little. I do not understand how it is that I do not gain, whilst my condition otherwise seems to improve and my appetite is comparatively good. I am afraid the cough and trouble will come back when cold weather sets in, since whenever after a rain it is chilly I feel this tickling sensation in the throat.

These are the symptoms and my condition in few words. What have you to say as to my condition?

Thanking you for your kindness,
    Yours truly,
        Rev. Fr. Henry J. Ehr.

Elgin, Ill., April 3, '97.

Mr. W. J. Clancy—*Dear Sir:*

Your treatment is strengthening me not only in lungs but in every way, and has proven a wonderful aid to digestion.

Six months ago physicians advised me to leave this climate on account of my lungs. Today physicians who know nothing of your treatment, pronounce my lungs clear and sound, and my friends remark daily my improved color and strength.

I feel that I cannot speak too highly of what you have done for me, and should anyone refer to me shall cheerfully recommend your treatment.

With a reasonable trial I am sure they will find it satisfactory.

    Sincerely yours,

      LOUIS L. STEVENS,
    478 Laurel St., Elgin, Ill.

July 1, 1898.

Pittsburgh Railway Co., Relief Dept.—W. J. CLANCY—*Dear Sir:*

I have just got home from my vacation, and will give you a brief synopsis of my cases:

Case I. The young lady is doing well. Was over this A. M. She complains only of pains in her limbs. Has some cough. Temperature and pulse normal. Appetite fine.

Case II. Old gentleman with Bright's disease has quit taking the medicine, as he says he does not need it.

Case III. Young lady at Ravenna is going to Cleveland to spend the 4th. Needs no explanation.

Case IV. Young man has had two hemorrhages before beginning treatment. I have not seen him since I have returned, but do not anticipate much improvement.

Case V. Young man in Cleveland has gained eight pounds in about three weeks. Needs no comments.

Case VI. Old gentleman with Bright's disease. Have not seen him since returning home.

Case VII. Master Car Builder's daughter in Allegheny. Have not heard from her.

Case VIII. Motorman. Tried the medicine three weeks. His wife came up last night and took half month's treatment.

Yours truly,
W. B. MIDDLETON, M. D.
Cuyahoga Falls, Ohio.

Chicago, Ill, April 16, 1897.

MR. CLANCY—*Dear Sir:*

Last May I was suffering with rheumatism, and was so crippled that I had to walk on crutches. I put myself under the St. Philip's Special Remedies Co., and with one week's treatment I was free from pain, and had no more use for the crutches. Since that time I have been in good health.

Yours respectfully,

WALTER O'CONNOR.

625 Flournay St.

Durango, Col., July 8, 1898.

MR. CLANCY—*St. Philip's Special Remedies Company, Chicago, Ill.—Dear Sir:*

I feel better in every respect, and while I am not rid of the catarrh yet, I have none of the symptoms that precede hay fever, and as this is about the time for it to commence I don't believe I will have it this year.

I will not miss an opportunity to recommend your treatment.

> Very respectfully,
> GEO WEAVER,
> La Plata County, Durango, Col.

Department of Police, August, 1898.—St. Philip's Special Remedies Company, 1412-1413 Masonic Temple. Gentlemen:
Being troubled with both muscular and inflammatory rheumatism for fourteen years (14 yrs.), part of the time being unable to get out of bed.

A friend of mine recommended Clancy Discoveries for Rheumatism, etc., and after using for about three months I received a perfect cure.

I would indorse it to any one troubled with such diseases, etc.

> Respectfully,
> ARTHUR CONNOLLY,
> Office at 27th Precinct Station, Chicago, or 304 S. Leavite St., City.

Chicago, Ill., Dec. 8, 1898.

MR. CLANCY—*Dear Sir:*

On June 15, 1898, I was taken with a severe hemorrhage while at work, and was forced to leave and hardly able to get home, having had three before that date inside of three weeks; lost 25 pounds in weight inside of a month, and had no appetite. I was examined by our family physician, Dr. C. H. Lovewell, [(R.) 6058 Wentworth ave., Med'l Dept. Univ. Mich., '71, Cor. Sec. Union Med'l Soc., Mem. Ill. State Med'l Soc.] I was informed by him that I had tuberculosis of the lungs, and advised to leave this climate immediately, as there was no hope for me in medicine.

I heard from a friend of the Clancy treatment, so decided I'd try it, not having any faith in it at the time, and inside of three months I was well, and am working hard every day, and gained twenty-two pounds.

Yours respectfully,

J. A. HOWARD.

5902 Butler St., Chicago, Ill.

Allegheny, Pa., May 25, 1898.

Mr. W. J. Clancy, *Room 1412-13 Masonic Temple, Chicago, Ill.—Dear Sir:*

On my return home I found my daughter in a very critical condition. Her limbs are badly swollen, and on consulting Dr. Hardtmeyer, advises me that he has called in other doctors into consultation and they know of no remedy that will possibly save her. I have arranged with him to make a thorough diagnosis of her case and forward same to you with full letter of explanation in her case. I understand from him that his examination shows tube casts and that he has no hope whatever.

Now, Mr. Clancy, if there is any possible way that you can use your remedies in this case I want you to do it without sparing any expense. If you think that you would understand the case more thoroughly, or it would do any good to have you come and see her, would be pleased to have you do so, and I will pay all expenses. If there is any springs or anything of that nature in the United States that you know of that would be beneficial in connection with your remedies, would be pleased to have you advise me so I can arrange to have her taken there.

Watch for the letter from Dr. Hardtmayer, aad as soon as you receive it go to work on it as quickly as possible, as it may be very dangerous to delay. The only hopes in the world I have of saving her life is in your remedies, and I do not wish you to spare any expense or trouble in connection with this matter.

Let me hear from you as soon as possible, and if necessary use the wire.

Yours truly,

W. J. BURKE.

Allegheny, Pa., May 25, 1898.

To MR. W. J. CLANCY, Chicago.—*Dear Sir:*

Mr. W. J. Burke of this city requests me to write to you about his daughter's case. Miss Burke has been ill for the last two years, suffering from Bright's disease. I have attended her for about two months, and during said time her urine has been constantly laden with albumen and tube casts. Dropsy also existed during the time that I attended her, and is now more marked than ever. Have given her all the treatment that I found to be beneficial in such cases, but thus far failed to do her any good. Mr. Burke seems to have great faith in a remedy that you possess, I therefore wish you would write to Mr. Burke and also send him some medicine if you think best. Any help you may be able to bestow upon the young lady in question will be fully appreciated by

Yours respectfully.

H. R. HARDTMAYER, M. D.

Chicago, Ill., May 27, 1898.

H. R. HARDTMAYER, M. D., 132 Liberty St., Allegheny, Pa.—*Dear Doctor:*

In reply to your very favored letter of the 25th inst., contents of same have been carefully noted.

Doctor, I would be pleased if you would inform me as to the amount of urine voided in each twenty-four hours, also specific gravity.

I would also be pleased to have you inform me the extent of this dropsical condition, and the condition of the heart, or has the child up to the present shown any signs of uræmic poisoning? If not I think my remedies may possibly be of some benefit to her. Any information you give me regarding this case will be considered a personal favor by me.

Doctor, should you deem it necessary, you can give saline cathartics in connection with my remedies, also any of the potash salts, as the above will not have any deleterious effect on the action of my medicine.

Trusting to hear from you as soon as convenient, I remain,

Very respectfully,

W. J. CLANCY.

Chicago, Ill., May 27, 1898.

W. J. BURKE, ESQ., 29 Resaco St., Allegheny, Pa.—*Dear Sir:*

In reply to your favored letter of the 25th inst., I have noted it very carefully, also received letter from Dr. Hardmayer this A. M., and I am sorry to know that the doctor has given up all hope; he also said your daughter has had dropsy for over two months, and that it is more marked now than before, as a consequence of this it must leave the heart in a very weak condition, and I can not give the medicine in as strong a dose as I would like to; but still I believe your daughter has a chance and I will send two bottles of medicine to you for her at once.

The black medicine is to be given in teasponful doses; it is compounded expressly for her, and the directions are on the bottle; one teaspoonful three times daily; for two days give it only twice a day, then wire me and I will reply. I also sent you a bottle of light medicine. It is especially adapted to relieve the cough, and it will reduce pains and relieve the breathing; also helps the bowels and removes dizziness. The directions call for half teaspoonful twice a day; it is not necessary to take that medicine regular, unless the above symptoms should require it.

Be sure and have the attending physician see that the bowels move freely; it will keep the swelling down.

Write me for a week every day, and if necessary to make change in doses of medicine, I will do so by wire.

It is not necessary for me to go to Allegheny, but trust that the medicine which I have forwarded will help her.

WM. J. CLANCY.

Chicago, Ill., May 27, 1898.
(Telegram.)

Posta. Telegraph—Cable Company.

WILLIAM J. BURKE, 29 Resaco St., Allegheny, Pa.:

I received your special delivery, also Dr. Hardtmayer's letter; will send you medicine at once; instructions will follow.

WM. J. CLANCY.

Allegheny, Pa., May 29, 1898.

MR. W. J. CLANCY—*Rooms 1412-1413 Masonic Temple Bldg., Chicago.*—*Dear Sir:*

Received the medicine O. K., and the doctor started to give it to Mamie at 10 o'clock this morning. She is some better than she was. Her throat is still quite sore. Yours respectfully,

W. J. BURKE.

Pittsburg, Pa., May 31, 1898.
(*Telegram.*)

Western Union Telegraph Company.

MR. CLANCY—*1412 Masonic Temple, Chicago:*

Daughter much better; swelling reduced; pulse strong; heart action good; giving three teaspoonfuls a day.

W. J. BURKE.

Pittsburg, Pa., May 31, 1898.

MR. CLANCY, *Chicago, Ill.—Dear Sir:*

We have been giving your remedy to my daughter since Sunday morning at 10 o'clock as directed, viz., a teaspoonful three times a day, and am more than pleased to be able to write you that she is today very much improved.

Her pulse is very much stronger and the heart action is very good, and the swelling has gone down considerable.

The doctor is going to make a test on her urine tomorrow for albumen, and day after tomorrow I will write you again, giving results of this test.

We will continue with the three teaspoonfuls a day until I hear from you.

Yours truly,

W. J. BURKE.

Chicago, Ill., June 1, 1898.
(*Telegram.*)
Postal Telegraph Company.

W. J. BURKE, *29 Resaco St., Allegheny, Pa.:*
Your daughter on fair way to recovery; continue medicine three times daily.

WM. J. CLANCY.

Pittsburg, Pa., June 2, 1898.

MR. W. J. CLANCY, *Chicago, Ill.—Dear Sir:*
My daughter still continues to improve, and today has some color in her ears; but

her appetite is not good yet, and she is yet bothered with pains in her legs and arms.

Please advise me if we shall begin to give her the white medicine, and oblige,

Yours truly,
W. J. BURKE.

Chicago, Ill., June 4, 1898.

(*Telegram.*)

WM. J. BURKE, 29 Resaco St., Allegheny, Pa

Give your daughter of the light medicine half teaspoonful twice a day. It will relieve the pains. I am pleased to note improvement.

W. J. CLANCY.

Western Union Telegraph Co.

Pittsburgh, Pa., June 3, 1898.

W. J. CLANCY, Room 1412 Masonic Temple, Chicago:

Daughter still improving. Doctor finds one-third less albumen.

W. J. BURKE.

9:24 P. M.

Pittsburgh, Pa., June 7, 1898.
(*Telegram.*)

Mr. W. J. Clancy, Chicago, Ill., *Dear Sir:*

My little girl is up and very much better. She has very good appetite and I think is going to be entirely cured.

W. J. Burke.

Chicago, Ill, June 9, 1898.

W. J. Burke, Allegheny, Pa.—*Dear Sir:*

In reply to your favored letter of the 8th inst., contents of same were carefully noted. I am pleased to note that your daughter is improving and is able to be up and feeling good, but be careful and do not give only liquid food to her, as her stomach is weak and unable to digest solid food, and should solid food be partaken of is liable to cause an attack of indigestion which would be far worse than her nephrites condition. I think your daughter will improve rapidly and eventually regain her health and strength. Trusting you will inform me regularly, so I can meet any irregularities that may arise.

W. J. Clancy.

Chicago, Ill., June 9, 1898.
(*Telegram.*)

W. J. BURKE, 29 Resaco St., Allegheny, Pa.—

Letter received. Be careful and only give daughter liquid food for some time.

WM. J. CLANCY.

Pittsburgh, Pa., June 10, 1898.

W. J. CLANCY, ESQ , Chicago.—*Dear Sir:*

Answering your valuable favor of the 8th inst., I informed the nurse who is taking care of my little daughter of your instructions, also gave the doctor the same information.

The doctor thinks a little solid food would not hurt her; but I told the nurse not to give her anything but liquid food for a few days, until I heard from you again.

She is improving very fast, and the doctor allowed her to go down stairs today. The doctor says he is almost ready to take his hat off to the treatment.

Thanking you very much for the great interest you have taken in my daughter's case, and especially for the careful and prompt attention given.

I am, truly yours,
W. J. BURKE.

Chicago, June 14, 1898.
(*Telegram.*)

WM. J. BURKE, 29 Resaco St., Allegheny, Pa.:

Letter received. Medicine shipped by today's express.

WM. J. CLANCY.

Allegheny, Pa., June 13, 1898.

W. J. CLANCY, Masonic Temple, Chicago, Ill.—*Dear Sir:*

Had a talk with Dr. Hardtmayer today in regard to condition of my daughter. He says her temperature is normal, her respiration good, and her general condition wonderfully improved; her appetite is good and she is improving fast as possible.

There is only enough medicine to last about three days. Please send another supply, as I would not want her to run out for the world. Urine shows that about two-thirds of the albumen has disappeared.

W. J. BURKE.

Chicago, Ill., June 15, 1898.

W. J. BURKE, ESQ., *29 Resaco St., Allegheny, Pa.—Dear Sir:*

In reply to your favored letter of the 13th inst., contents were carefully noted. Was pleased to note your daughter's improvement, and believe the child is out of danger. Do not give solid food for ten days or two weeks. and then only sparingly.

Please request the attending nurse to instruct your daughter how to practice deep breathing, so as to develop the chest, as it is necessary to breath as much air as possible by each respiration of the lungs.

I will explain the means by which the respiratory movements are affected, the inspiratory muscles engaged in ordinary inspiration are the diaphragm, the external intercostal, the levatores costarum and seratus posticus superior, the vertical diameter of the chest to increase by the contraction and consequently descent of the diaphragm, the sides of the muscles descending most and the central tendon remaining comparatively unmoved, while the intercostal and other muscles by acting at the same time prevent the diaphragm during its contraction from drawing in the sides of the chest.

If you will have the nurse follow my instructions and practice the abdominal breathing as above, you will soon note the rosy cheeks of your daughter, which will be caused by the amount of oxygen in the blood, which increased the red corpuscles, as it is positively known that oxygen is not in simple solution of the blood, but is contained in the red corpuscles of the blood. Of course judgment must be used and not overdo the instructions.

W. J. CLANCY.

Pittsburgh, June 25, 1898.

To Mr. W. J. Clancy, Chicago.—*Dear Sir:*

Doctor Hardtmayer called to see my daughter yesterday and said she was improving fast as could be expected, but there is still some albumen and tube casts. She is looking very good and able to be up and around, and was down to the park yesterday.

We are not allowing her any solid food and the nurse is putting her through the exercise per your instructions.

There are a great many people here watching this case.

W. J. BURKE.

Allegheny, Pa., June 29, 1898.

W. J. Clancy, Esq., Chicago, Ill.—*Dear Sir:*

My daughter is nearly out of medicine again. She appears to be getting along nicely, and is anxious to know when she can commence to eat solid food.

W. J. BURKE.

Chicago, Ill., June 30, 1898.

W. J. BURKE, ESQ., 29 Resaco St., Allegheny, Pa.—*Dear Sir:*

Yours of the 28th inst. at hand and contents noted. I will send you a bottle of medicine for your daughter; same strength as she has been taking. I do not know when it would be best for your daughter to partake of solid food, but I feel as though it is too soon yet; still you can have the attending physician decide. You see I can only judge by cases I treated which was in same condition your daughter was in when I took up the case. Of course if it was so I could see the child I might think different, and in fact suggest solid food diet; but as it is I am apprehensive and feel safe to know that only liquid foods are partaken of. I wish you would write the amount of urine voided during the night, also the amount during the day; also specific gravity, the color if possible; also if increasing in weight; her present weight, and weight six months back if possible.

Trusting to hear from you more frequently about the child, I remain,

W. J. CLANCY.

Pittsburgh, Pa., July 27, 1898.

Mr. W. J. Clancy, Chicago, Ill.—*Dear Sir:*

Am pleased to be able to inform you that my little daughter continues to improve. Will you kindly send me another bottle of the medicine, as there is only a little left in the bottle, and my wife thinks that it has begun to sour, and oblige,

Yours truly,

W. J. Burke.

Allegheny, Pa., Sept. 30, 1898.

W. J. Clancy, Chicago, Ill.—*Dear Sir:*

I yesterday made an analysis of Miss Burke's urine and to my astonishment found the same perfectly normal; albumen and casts having entirely disappeared. She is improving daily.

Will you kindly instruct me if you consider it necessary to continue the medicine, and if so will you please forward a new supply, as she is entirely out of the same. In hopes that I may soon hear from you, I remain, with best wishes,

Yours respectfully,

Dr. H. R. Hardtmayer.

Pittsburgh, Pa., Oct. 27, 1898.

[Information for Medical and Surgical Register.—Name: Han's R. Hardtmayer. Residence: 132 Liberty St., Allegheny, Pa. Graduation: Jefferson Medical, Philadelphia, 1877. Degree: M. D. Appointments: Physician for the Pittsburgh and Western Railroad; Medical Examiner German Life Insurance Company, New York. Medical Societies, member of: Allegheny County and State Medical.]

The above Han's R. Hardtmayer, M. D., prescribed the treatment in this case, and also pronounced the young girl free of all traces of her former trouble, viz: Bright's Disease.

Chicago, Ill., May 26, 1897.

MR. CLANCY—*Dear Sir:*

It affords me very great pleasure to be able to state to you that my case of Bright's disease, for which I was treated by a number of prominent physicians, without success, has so far progressed that I can safely state to you that I feel in a short time I will be entirely cured of my trouble. I cannot say too much of your method of treatment for my particular disease and have no hesitancy in recommending it to anyone suffering from the same.

Very respectfully,

HENRY SEGER,

241 W. Monroe St., Chicago.

Chicago, Ill., Oct. 20, 1898.

MR. CLANCY—*Dear Sir:*

I write you these few lines to express my thanks for my recovery from Bright's disease through the agency of your treatment, as I had treated with the very best physicians in Chicago without any benefit. I am now able to follow my trade, as a painter, for the last twelve months, and feel entirely well. You can use this letter as you see fit.

Yours respectfully,

HENRY SEGER.

241 W. Monroe St., Chicago.

[Specialists: Hoodley, M. D., Mitchell Cliford, M. D., Isaac N. Danforth, M. D. Seger was treated by above Specialists. Insured in Prudential Insurance Co. Since been *cured*.]

[The above Henry Seger has since been granted a life insurance in one of our leading insurance companies. He is in perfect health and is in charge of a gang of painters, in the employ of G. J. McCarthy, painter and decorator, located in the City of Chicago, State of Illinois.]

Chicago, Ill., Sept. 1, 1898.

Mr. Clancy:

I want to thank you for all that you have done for me, also to let others suffering as I was from Bright's disease know what your medicine will do. Some of the best doctors in Chicago told me I had but a short time to live, by dieting, and that there was no cure for me, because no medicine could reach the kidneys. I suffered terribly, and even though I was on a diet I didn't get any better. I heard of your medicine from those that had been cured, and thought that I would try it. After taking it three days I gave up dieting and could eat the same as the rest of the family, and now, after two years, I have had no return of the trouble.

Anyone wishing any more particulars I will be only too pleased to give them by addressing me at 131 South Albany Ave., Chicago.

Very respectfully,
Mary E. O'Connor.

Chicago, Ill, Dec. 12, 1898.

St. Philip's Special Remedies Company,
1412 Masonic Temple—*Gentlemen:*

I am pleased to be able to testify to the great success obtained by my wife for the cure effected upon her for tuberculosis of the kidneys and bladder, with the use of Clancy's Discoveries, and many a time of late my wife and family thank you for the great cure wrought in her case, when our family physician, one of the best on the South Side of the city as well as the best physicians in one of our hospitals here, could do nothing for her, and in fact classed her case as incurable.

She was taken down with the dreaded disease in August, and after doctoring a few weeks at home without any success, she was induced to go to the hospital.

The physicians there had her urine diagnosed and found tuberculosis bacilli, and they undertook to treat her for the disease, but at the end of three weeks she was worse than when she entered the place and the irritation and spasmodic pains she suffered were telling on her fast and she could not have withstood the strain much longer so I took her home again, believing that she was growing worse under their treatment.

After the second week at home she began to grow very weak, and the spasms after urinating became more frequent, and we began to dispair of her recovery.

About this time a friend of ours, who was cured by your remedy for tuberculosis of the lungs, urged me to try your treatment for my wife's ailment and I consented to do so.

I had a second diagnosis of her case made before commencing your treatment with the following result: specific gravity of the urine 10.10 tuberculosis bacilli in the urine; heart very weak and constitution greatly run down.

Another examination on the third week showed specific gravity 10.15, or normal, for a person of her age and weight; the bacilli very scanty and small; heart stronger and a general improvement in her condition.

In November I had three examinations made with the following results: Specific gravity of urine 10.15; tuberculosis bacilli entirely absent; her heart in its usual normal condition and a noticeable change for the better generally.

About the first week in November she began to walk without help, before which time she had to be carried from one place to another, being almost helpless in her lower extremities.

She is now able to be up and around and is improving rapidly; sleeps well, eats well and feels remarkably well for one who has so recently gone through such great exhaustion and suffering.

She will be glad to be interviewed by any one concerning her case and the wonderful cure effected on her by your remedies.

I must not forget to mention that she commenced with your treatment on Sept. 27th, and that after the second week she began to experience a decided improvement in her condition.

Hoping this testimonial of your remedies for the cure of tuberculosis will have the effect I earnestly desire it to have, at least upon any person similarly afflicted, as was my wife, I remain,

Yours very truly,

L. D. MANNIX, 4006 Wabash Ave.

I was treated by Dr. Byron S. Turner, (R.), Chi. Med'l, 1878; Mem, Am. Med'l Assn., and Ill. State Med'l Soc., E., he being our family physician.

Was treated in Baptist Hospital by Dr. Linnie Owsley, who had microscopical analysis made of urine at the Columbus Laboratory, the same showed tuberculosis bacilli.

Previous examinations made by Dr. Byron S. Turner showed tuberculosis bacilli in sputum.

[Dr. Linnie M. Owsley; H., 3410 Rhodes Ave.; Hahn., Chi., '90; Res. Supt. and Att'g Obstet'n Chi. Baptist Hosp.; Supt. Baptist Hosp. Training School for Nurses; Mem. Ill. Homo. Med'l Assn., L.]

The latter microscopical analysis were made by Dr. D. J. Carey with the following results: "Urine in 24 hours, 40 ounces; specific gravity, 10.15; light straw color; free of puss; slightly acid; no disagreeable odor; and I failed to find any evidence of tuberculosis bacilli after several tests on three different miscroscopical analysis."

Yours, very respectfully,
MRS. L. D. MANNIX,
4006 Wabash Ave.

PUBLISHER'S AFFIDAVIT.

Chicago, Ill., Dec. 16, 1898.

John A. Kutz, publisher of "Manifesto of Plain Facts by Wm. J. Clancy, M. C., and D. J. Carey, M. D.," being first duly sworn, on oath says, that the foregoing letters of testimonials are printed from original letters and are true in every case.

STATE OF ILLINOIS } ss.
COOK COUNTY.

I, F. E. Bartlett, a Notary Public in and for said State and County, do certify that the said John A. Kutz appeared personally before me and acknowledges the above to be true in every particular. F. E. BARTLETT,
[SEAL.] Notary Public.
Dated this 16th day of December, 1898.

CONCLUSION.

Dear Friends:

IN CONCLUSION we would ask: Has it ever occurred to you the amount of space usually required or alloted to a bed chamber? The average space is 8x8x9--576 cubic feet or 995.328 cubic inches. An adult confined in a bed chamber requires and breaths 600 cubic inches of air each minute. In twenty-four hours approximately the square of the air contained in this bed chamber has been through the respiratory organs of the tubercular patient. In other words, the air has circulated throughout the apartments and as a consequence the air must be impregnated with bacilli. This condition exists to a greater or less degree throughout the course of the disease.

Now we come to the family physician who has treated the patient since childhood, and as a consequence the patient places entire confidence in the physician. The physician understanding this, also knowing the patient has only a short time to live, feels that he should not loose this confidence and tries to console and make the patient as comfortable as possible. To do this he must remain with the patient for at least thirty minutes. During his visit he has approximately breathed 20,000 cubic inches of the air which is actually one-fourth laden with parasites of tubercular bacilli. This physician, being a prominent one, he has a number of such cases, oftentimes having three or four such patients to visit each twenty-four hours. In all cases such advice and council has been given willingly. This physician has practiced medicine in great many cases from thirty to fifty years, and year after year attended tubercular patients as above stated and still is in perfect health. Not one symptom of tuberculosis ever troubled him. How so? The physician is a model man, regular and moderate in all his habits, pays particular attention to his stomach and partakes of such nurishment that agrees with him; also is cautious in not over stimulating it by drugs or by stimulants. He uses water plentifully both internally and externally, the one and only absolute stimulant given by God unadulterated. Hence healthy assimulation. The lungs are bacillicidal, and being supplied with healthy, transformed food into such a neutrient condition that it is taken up by the circulatory system to form an integral part of the economy. The secondary change taking place in the lungs is the conversion of food into blood by the chemical action that is constantly going on in the lungs. The oxygen consuming the carbon also consumes all bacteria and other parasites that may be inhaled post natal or partaken in solid or in liquid form. Therefore tuberculosis is a constitutional disease and is not caused from inhalation of the bacilli, nor from foods. If persons are in fair health, and especially their stomach, they can ingest a quart of the bacilli every twenty-four hours and they would not affect them in the least, no more than they affected the physician who has been breathing them as freely as he knew how for fifty years and still has no fear of them.

The medical colleges and practicing physicians have for all times opposed nostrums and inhalation treatments for the cure of pulmonary tuberculosis. Why? First, because physiologically speaking the theory of calling consumption a local disease is against the established doctrines of medicine, and can not be true without overturning the very foundation on which every physican's practice and reputation are based.

It is evident for years that the physicians thoroughly knew what was to be treated, but lacked the proper formula to compound the medicine that they chose to administer in such cases, and have been patiently waiting for the chemist to prepare it. Through William J. Clancy, a chemist, a formula has been brought to their notice that has been admistered under their instructions and has positively cured hundreds of well-developed cases of tuberculosis of the lungs, and now hail the perfection of their cherished hopes and hundreds of physicians are now using it in their practice.

The physicians referred to in the introduction of this book are in the minority and are the black sheep of the flock. They are as a rule in the profession to make money by hook or by crook. Not so with the majority of physicians. They have chosen the profession that is one of the noblest sacrifices that any one could undertake for the benefit of his fellow man. The doctor of today jeopardizes his health far oftener than the soldier on the battlefield. He has not an hour or minute that he can call his own, and few there are, I dare say, that follow their vocation as physicians who are doing so for mercenary ends. Of course there are a few exceptions.

The Chicago Chronicle, Tuesday morning, Nov. 29, 1898, published the following article, and I agree with the writer that through the scare caused by known germs that we are neglecting the cause that is producing the trouble. For centuries consumption has been prevalent, known as decline.

Now, should consumption be hereditary and contagious, as some are supposed to believe, there would not be any living persons today.

A local physician of ability, discussing the death at San Juan, Porto Rico, of Mr. George S. Willits, attributes that gentleman's death to lockjaw, which, he says, is caused by the microbe of tetanus. But in speaking further of the matter he declares that "death from lockjaw is frequently caused by exhaustion and failure of the heart muscles." The statements are not reconcilable. Tetanus is either caused by a microbe or it is not. The bacteriological theory must cover all cases or none of them. And the same thing is true of other germ diseases so called. The bacteriological experts agree that we are daily exposed to germs of all kinds—tuberculosis, pneumonia, and even diphtheria, yet a relatively small percentage of mankind succumb to those diseases daily. The reason given is that only a small percentage of those exposed are susceptible, which sounds like giving up the whole case. If the "bugs" are innocuous to 99 per cent. of those exposed it looks as though the illness of the remaining 1 per cent. might as well be attributed to some cause other than bacterial infection. The fact that the bacilli of tuberculosis, for instance, are invariably found in the sputum of consumptives doesn't necessarily prove that the bacilli caused consumption. May they not be the effect of it? Some people think so, and it is significant that the "bug" theory has helped therapeutics mighty little in dealing with pneumonia and la grippe, for instance. Doctors did quite as well when the former disease was known as "lung fever" and the latter as a "bad cold."

INDEX.

	PAGES.
Acute Gout	168 to 172
Acute Rheumatism	157 to 162
Bright's Disease	139 to 143
Chronic Gout	173 to 175
Chronic Rheumatism	165 to 166
Conclusion	306 to 311
Diet, Hints on	200 to 219
Essentials on Bacteriology	84 to 94
Erythema	145 to 149
Erysipelas	151 to 155
Liquids	239 to 246
Newspaper Investigations	177 to 198
Preface	2 to 12
Physiology	13 to 79
Pulmonary Tuberculosis	107 to 115
Pneumonia	117 to 128
Publisher's Affidavit	305
Scrofula	96 to 105
Sciatic Rheumatism	164
Tuberlosis Bacilli	81 to 82
Testimonials	248 to 304
Vegetable Food	221 to 237
What Constitutes Bright's Disease	130 to 137

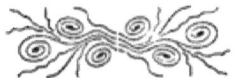

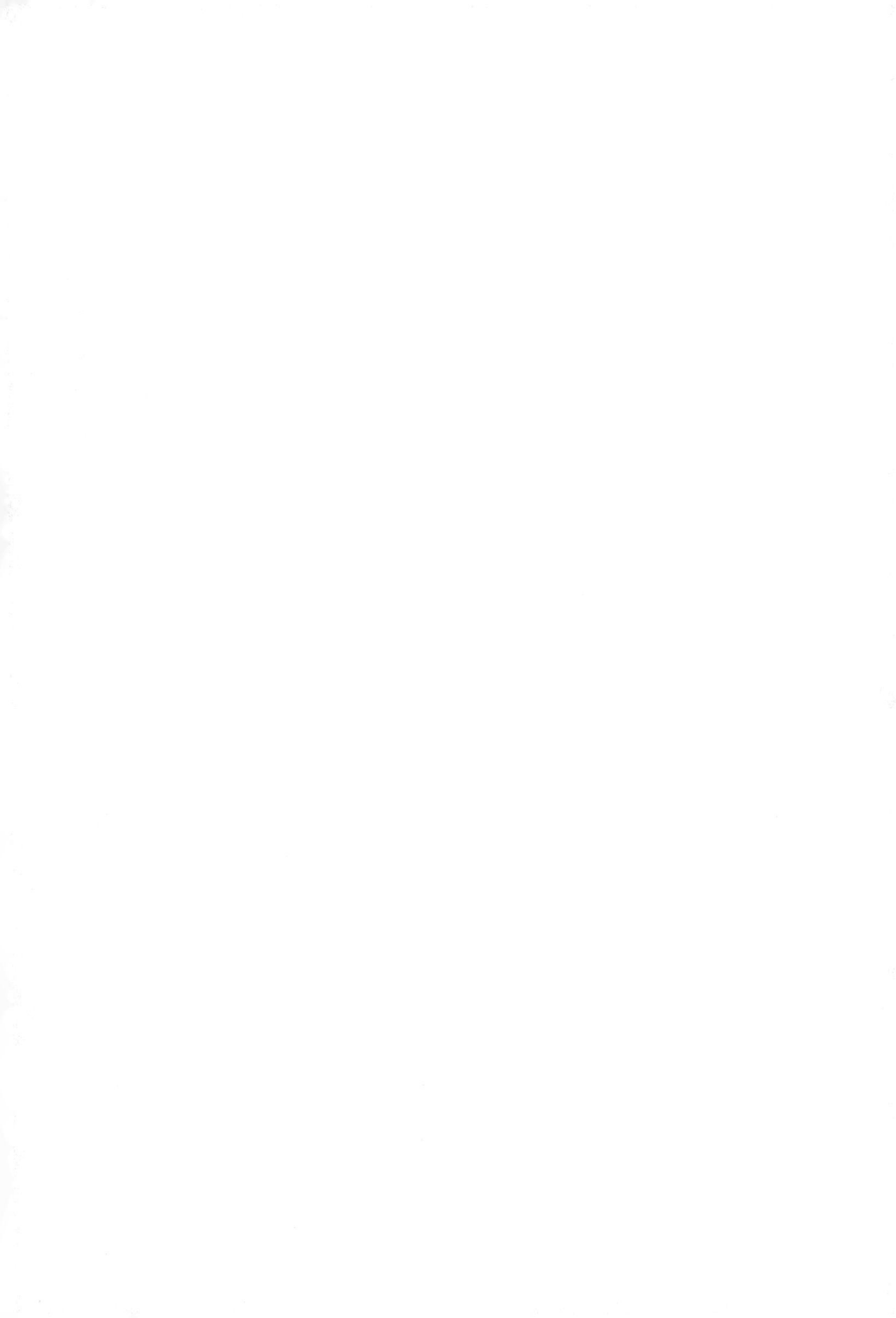

www.ingramcontent.com/pod-product-compliance
Lightning Source LLC
Chambersburg PA
CBHW030808230426
43667CB00008B/1117